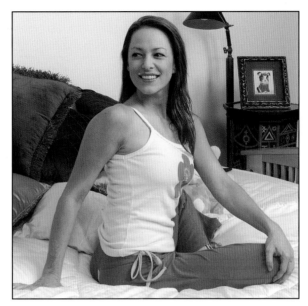

YOGA in BED

YOGA in BED

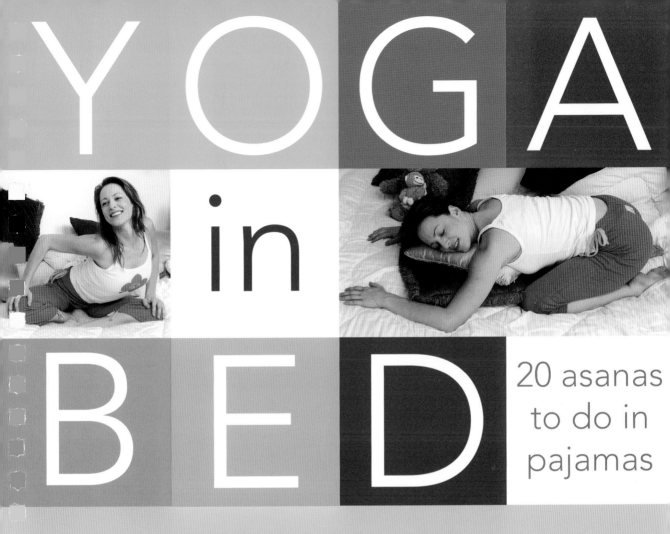

BED

20 asanas
to do in
pajamas

by Edward Vilga

RUNNING PRESS
PHILADELPHIA · LONDON

For all of my teachers and students,
each of whom has inspired me along the way.

© 2005 by Edward Vilga
All rights reserved under the Pan-American and International Copyright Conventions
Printed in the United States

This book may not be reproduced in whole or in part, in any form or by any means, electronic or mechanical, including photocopying, recording, or by any information storage and retrieval system now known or hereafter invented, without written permission from the publisher

9 8 7 6 5 4 3 2 1

Digit on the right indicates the number of this printing

Library of Congress Control Number: 2004096954

ISBN 0-7624-2341-2

Cover and interior design by Corinda Cook
Edited by Deborah Grandinetti
Photo Shoot directed by Edward Vilga
All photography by David Plakke (www.davidplakke.com), except photo on page 104 © Corbis Royalty-free
Model: Cristy Candler
Typography: Avenir and Baskerville

This book may be ordered by mail from the publisher. Please include $2.50 for postage and handling.
But try your bookstore first!

Running Press Book Publishers
125 South Twenty-second Street
Philadelphia, Pennsylvania 19103-4399

Visit us on the web!
www.runningpress.com

Contents

Disclaimer

Although the yoga poses in this book are designed to be gentle and appropriate for almost everyone, the author and publisher advise readers to know their physical limits and take full responsibility for their well-being. As with any exercise program, get your doctor's approval before beginning.

If you have lower back pain, be sure to consult your physician or a certified yoga instructor before beginning an at-home practice. If you get the okay and you decide to try these postures, be very attentive to your spine. One lower-back modification that tends to be helpful for all lying-down poses, is to place a rolled up blanket or several pillows beneath the knees.

Finally, many of the postures in this book are not appropriate for pregnant women. It is beyond the scope of this book to give variations for pregnancy. Yoga during pregnancy can be a provide a wonderful work-out, though and many other excellent yoga books can be found on this topic.

Preface

People often ask how *Yoga in Bed* came about.

After I became a yoga teacher, I began teaching some large classes, but I concentrated on private students. I love working one-to-one because it allows me to really focus on an individual and truly teach, something that's difficult to do in a mixed level gym class with 60 students, half of whom have drifted in for the day because Cardio Funk was full.

At the Laughing Lotus Yoga Center in New York City, I teach a free-wheeling, open level vinyasa class (coordinated breath and movement; like life, always changing and always challenging). Vinyasa-style yoga is joyful, highly charged stuff. It makes hard-core yogi athletes drip with sweat.

Yet as a private teacher, I found myself dealing with the very stiff, people for whom touching their toes was a distant dream. Frankly, they acknowledged they were more likely to reach Mars on the space shuttle than feel fingers connecting to their feet. These were not the select, small audience for my Vinyasa class; this was most of America: willing, eager to learn, but totally inflexible.

At the same time, teaching so steadily, I'd often not have time for a thorough practice of my own. In fact, when I was struggling to establish myself as a teacher, like many people launching careers, my life got super-hectic. There were weeks where every morning I'd awaken at 5AM, teach two people by 9AM, teach a third, then run off to a group class, followed by a second wave of evening clients. I barely had time to shower and leave the house, returning to stumble (happily) into bed, much less complete my former rigorous yoga practice. Sometimes a few stretches in bed—not even a downward dog—were all I could manage before rushing out again.

More and more, I began to see the growing disparity between the public classes I taught and what most people could actually do. True, a handful of yogis were interested in the correct placement of their tailbone for extreme backbends like Scorpion. Yet in "real life" I was teaching sixty-year-old *New Yorker* editors how to hang over their straight legs or Tony-winning playwrights how to lie on their back supported by some pillows under the knees to relieve stress.

Meanwhile, I was often spending ten minutes between my snooze alarm's blasts quickly stretching in bed on arising (or during my afternoon nap) before zipping off to teach again.

Spinning around book ideas with Dana Flynn—the amazing founder of the Laughing Lotus Yoga Center in Manhattan where I trained and now teach—the slightly zany title of *Yoga in Bed* was born. We thought the title was fun and very catchy, but also discovered that there was real value here.

I realized that this was a yoga practice that might actually work for people.

Taken from my own shorthand morning stretches, here was the simplest possible introduction to yoga: one that could be done entirely in bed. It felt absolutely great and frankly it was all I had time for. Most importantly, it was accessible for almost everyone physically and at the same time, was leavened with a Laughing Lotus touch of humor. And thus, originating from the bed of an over-worked yoga teacher, *Yoga in Bed* was born.

The more I share it, the more the value of *Yoga in Bed* keeps growing clearer.

First and foremost, it's the ultimate in CONVENIENCE. Most people are wildly busy, over-stressed, and over-scheduled. Putting "Start Taking Yoga Classes" on top of a crowded To-Do List just adds one more task that— when push comes to shove—probably won't be accomplished.

Yoga in Bed offers some gentle stretches and guided meditations that easily fit into anyone's schedule. No traveling to class required. And not only can these simple poses and meditations be done in the comfort and privacy of your own home, they can also be accomplished without even leaving your bed.

Secondly, in this book it's my goal to make the practice of yoga ACCESSIBLE. I've selected poses and practices that are within the range of most healthy individuals. These are not "yoga tricks" like putting your foot behind your head that some yoga books celebrate. These are poses that anyone can do and enjoy.

Thirdly, yoga is about COMMITMENT. It's my hope that *Yoga in Bed* becomes the foundation for a steady, life-long practice. By setting the practice in bed, the commitment needed to open the body is made much easier.

Each morning and every night, you're already exactly where you need to be to practice yoga twice a day. Why not add a few more moments of breath and movement to the mix? Opening the body up takes time—it took years of stress to tighten you up in the first place!—but once again, since you know you're going to land in your bed every night and wake up every morning, you're more than halfway towards the commitment of showing up to practice.

Another way of looking at this is that the commitment's made easier because *Yoga in Bed* is so ORGANIC. In fact, this is the way animals practice their brand of yoga. Just watch your dog or cat awaken from a nap (or settle down for rest). Without fail, they enjoy a few luxurious stretches before embarking on any activity.

For us, *Yoga in Bed* stretches serve as a natural segue to either waking up in the morning or going to sleep at night. Rather than taking an artificial chunk out of your day, like going to a gym and pointlessly running on a treadmill, nothing could be more natural than some stretches like these before getting up or going to bed.

Again, you probably do some basic stretching anyway, and by lengthening the process for ten minutes or more, you can significantly increase your health benefits and peace of mind.

Finally, *Yoga in Bed* makes sense because it is nice to give your home—particularly your private space—a feeling of the SACRED. Framing your sleep-time with some breath, movement, and meditation allows you to strengthen those vital connections within yourself.

You'll be amazed at how mind, body, and heart open up and enrich your entire life with the regular, gentle, fun practice of *Yoga in Bed*.

Thanks to all my students and teachers, particularly:

Immense gratitude first and foremost to Dana Flynn, from whose brilliant original inspiration this book was born. It was Dana Flynn who, with Jasmine Tarkeshi, gave me the yoga training that changed my life. Dana's generous, wild spirit always inspires, and their Laughing Lotus is a gorgeous, joyful place to call Home. Yogadana, thanks for the wings!

Emma Sweeney for her faith in this project and in me, and for the joy of having her as an agent.

Deborah Grandinetti at Running Press for being such a dream to work with on this project. Here's to many more!

Stacey Lynn Brass, yoga colleague and teaching partner, for her wonderful friendship and support, and her input on this book.

Alnoor Kassam, for all his heartfelt contributions, personal and professional.

Rosemarie Bria (and Midgie), who opened their home to us as the location for our photo shoot. Painting of Midgie by Dorothy Theodora Bria.

Lisa Lori, for coming on board and making the journey that much more exciting.

My gorgeous in every way model Cristy Candler. Truly, she redefines "fabulous," carrying the word to new heights. I hope we spend the rest of our days re-shooting together.

Everyone who made the photo shoots happen—particularly David Plakke—your photos are as beautiful as you were a professional joy to work with. Great thanks to Adam Mastrelli, Autumn Saville, Anne Marie Bradley, Tom Hamilton, and Rachel Levine for their various contributions.

Shane Condino, elephant poet and yoga guinea pig.

Hillary Kelleher for reading a draft and offering dreamy comments.

All my clients, especially Richard Freundlich and Stephen Anderson, for introductions wide and far.

My great friends over the years who've enriched my creative and personal life in innumerable ways: especially Amy Adler, Nicole Bettauer, and Genevieve Lynch. A particular thanks to Leslie Lewis Sword who has demonstrated both friendship and artistic faith in me so consistently and with such generosity and kindness.

To new friends and partners who've brought fresh inspiration at to this point in the path: Jon Chaloner, Julie Hilden, Stephen Glass, Jude English, and Amanda Macklowe.

Roger Gonzalez, Beloved Brat, transit of Venus and sharer of Neptunian adventures.

Finally, to my family for their boundless support.

Introduction:
Yoga (or Yogurt) in Your Bed?

* Everything you always wanted to know about yoga but were afraid to ask

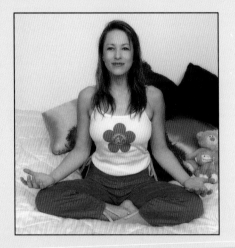

In this new millennium, everyone's heard about yoga, yet many people are still confused. Some people even wonder about the yoga/yogurt connection (there is none, both words just begin with "Yo").

So before I launch into the specifics of *Yoga in Bed*, here's some basic info about the Big Picture of what yoga is and how it can improve your life.

Exactly what is yoga? Is it a religion?

First of all, yoga is a philosophy, not a religion. It doesn't require adopting any new religious beliefs, just exploring the concepts of letting go, acceptance, and staying present. The goal of yoga according to the most ancient texts is "to calm the storms of the mind." In other words finding a quality of peace and happiness in our lives. That's a goal that's hard to argue with and of tremendous benefit to anyone.

So is yoga just doing poses like in a gym class?

No, yoga is far more than just physical poses. Although this is part of the practice, to really explore yoga means to not just stretch, but also to travel a highly ethical path, while pursuing breathing and centering meditation.

For many people, the physical practice is a first and major step. The body opens, and tensions start to dissolve in the muscles and the soul. But while just stretching is a very good thing, the universe of yoga—especially the possibility of finding more joy in your life—offers so much more.

What is the point of yoga poses?

The physical poses are designed to promote good health and release tension in the body so you can have a peaceful mind and a happy life. They have been perfected and adapted by many different yoga masters over the centuries so that almost anyone can approach them and derive tremendous health benefits.

How's it different from working out?

Yoga is not just another "work-out," however. It's not approached with a conventional work-out spirit. Teachers try to share the physical poses combined with the philosophical ideas of calming and centering. Good yoga classes encourage self-acceptance, non-competition, and gentleness in poses rather than pushing and getting aggressive.

Another major difference is that when practicing any pose, we're perhaps even more interested in what's going on inside the mind than we are in the body.

Correct alignment is absolutely important so that the mind/body connection will allow you to de-stress naturally. But perhaps more than this, slowing down and watching the breath allows you to develop a different, improved relationship with your own thoughts and feelings. In other words, the workout is both interior and exterior, physical and mental.

Who can do yoga?

Anyone, of any age or any fitness level. I've taught yoga to everyone from elementary school kids to retirees. All that's required is a willingness to learn (and have fun!)

There's no way I can ever get into some of those poses I see people doing.

Not everyone can do the same things, of course. It's important to know your limits. For example, if you have serious health problems, or lower back issues, or even if you're healthy and happily pregnant, than this book isn't necessarily right for you. Nonetheless, after speaking with your doctor and finding the right yoga instructor, there will definitely be some version of yoga that you can do.

As an example, standing on your head is a fantastic yoga pose, but not right for everyone. Most folks, however, can do UPSIDE DOWN RELAXATION (page 85) which offers many of the same benefits with far fewer challenges. Although seemingly miles apart from each other, the poses are both inversions that revitalize the system.

With a little creativity, and the right information, there will be a way to adapt any pose appropriately to exactly where you are right now.

Where does yoga come from?

Yoga originated over 5,000 years ago in India. The oldest writings—the Yoga Sutras and the Upanishads—date from this time.

Yet Yoga is not carved in stone. It is continuously evolving and growing with many different styles as people constantly develop and explore the practice.

So there are many different kinds of yoga?

Yes, there are many different styles and flavors. Although they all have things in common and poses usually overlap, classes might feel and look very different.

For example, some classes such as Ashtanga or Vinyasa move flowingly. They emphasize coordinating the breath while moving from pose to pose.

Others are Iyengar-influenced, and might involve holding only a handful of poses, focusing on detailed alignment and working extremely specifically.

Restorative classes use poses and props to let the body hold a shape and open very deeply and slowly. Several of our poses in the Evening section are restorative, allowing you to sample this style of yogic letting go.

There are yoga practices like Kundalini where certain types of vigorous breathing and simple repetitive motions are more strongly emphasized. There are even newer-style classes these days (like Bikram) taking place in heated rooms because some people feel that opens the muscles up.

And of course there are classes like Yoga Mamas or Yoga Seniors and those that address other specific health concerns.

Part of the beauty of yoga is that it is so highly adaptable. With a little exploration, you're bound to find the practice that really speaks best to you.

Why should I do yoga?

Yoga helps with:

- Flexibility

- Deep Relaxation

- Feeling "Centered"

- Strength Building

- Balance and Coordination

- Healing

- Happiness and general sense of well-being

These are things that can benefit anyone and everyone.

Particularly as we grow older, the physical practice of yoga helps us increase and sustain our flexibility, without some of the harsher side-effects of other workouts.

How long does it take to 'get good' at yoga?

"Getting Good" doesn't mean mastering difficult poses.

Someone can practice yoga for years, developing much greater health and peace of mind without ever bending themselves into a pretzel. Everyone is different, and all measures of progress have to be evaluated individually. While it's exciting to have students experience breakthroughs—today I touched my toes!—what's gratifying is the increased awareness they have of their bodies and an overall feeling of greater contentment in their lives. How long does this take? Even a single yoga session can teach you something about the body and the mind, although a steady practice is required to really get the greatest benefits. The most important thing is just getting started!

Morning Poses:

Invigorate

YOUR

AM

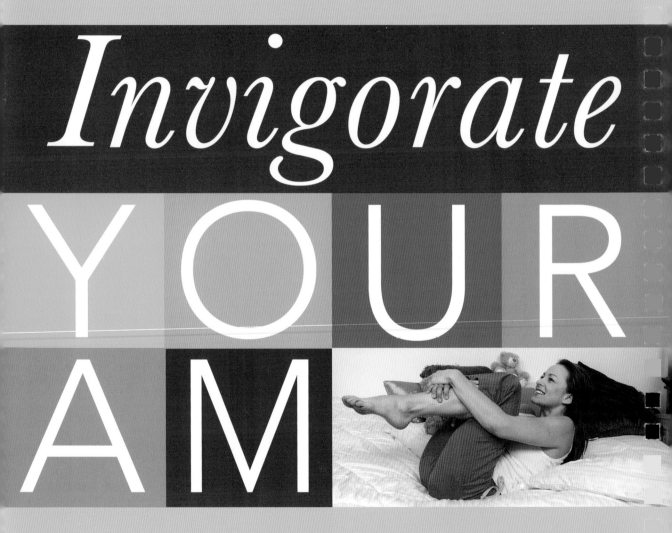

While doing yoga, you breathe through your nose.

Some people develop the bad habit of breathing through their mouths. There are indeed those days when a cold stuffs you up, so while this mouth-breathing won't kill you, you won't have all the great benefits that breathing through the nose provides.

The ideal way to breathe is to let the air come through the nostril, traveling all the way through the lungs and filling them up. When you inhale, you let go of all the muscles in the belly, so it's as if it fills up with air. Breathing in, belly expands. When you're nicely full—without any straining—simply release and exhale.

If you watch babies, you'll notice this is how they breathe. It's effortless and naturally sweet. Somehow as we grow older we lose track of this kind of simple, healthy pleasure.

Let *Yoga in Bed* reconnect you with the fullness of your breath and all the terrific benefits this provides body, mind, and spirit.

Swinging Into Motion

Everybody knows that yoga's about staying loose and going with the flow.

Same thing with the poses in this book.

I've put them in an order but this order doesn't have to be followed exactly. Mixing the poses up won't hurt you. And on any given day, you can freely decide to linger in a pose as long as it feels comfortable, or omit one if it's not feeling right.

What's key is that stretching and breathing become part of your daily routine—without becoming routine and boring. Consistency is definitely the most important thing.

A little every day is infinitely more effective than a single big burst of activity every once in a while.

That's why *Yoga in Bed* is such a doable program: every morning and evening you're already in bed. Simply add a few stretches with breathing to feel yourself limbering up.

Again, the program is designed to work for you as an individual. Ultimately, yoga is extremely personal. In that spirit, it's true that no teacher or book knows exactly how you feel inside your body. Therefore it's important to keep learning more about where you need to let go, and then find the best poses to achieve that.

So if something doesn't feel right, be sensible and go easy on yourself and try something else. A nice stretchy feeling is terrific, but no pose should ever come anywhere near hurting. There's bound to be a pose that feels great as it opens you up.

Most importantly, as you explore these poses, have fun along the way. Don't take them—or yourself—too seriously. As long as the feeling is peaceful and opening, trust that you're doing it right. In other words, just go with the flow, letting *Yoga in Bed* take you there.

Sunrise Stretch

Lift your hands above your head.
Inhale and stretch your fingers away from your toes.
Relax on the exhale, letting everything go.

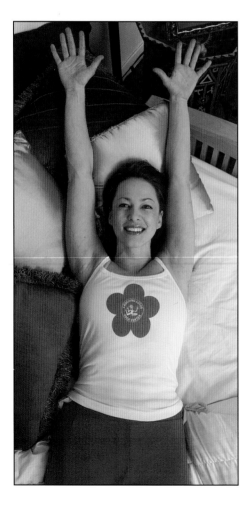

This simple stretch feels absolutely great. You're lengthening yourself in an easy, friendly way, waking up every part of your body.

Lying down, make sure your back feels comfortable. If it's acting up, keep a soft bend in the knees. Placing some pillows under the knees can also be soothing.

Lift your hands past your head, reaching the fingers away from the toes as you inhale.

As you exhale, you can release, letting everything get floppy.

Hang out here, repeating the stretchy inhale and the releasing exhale several times.

As you inhale, let your feet flex and the toes point away.

Really fill up with air—breathing through your nose—so that when you exhale and release everything, there might even be an audible sigh. Try this a handful of times to lengthen yourself and then release.

A few yawns or some deep sighing "Ahhhs" are also a great way to waken up the face and lungs. Adding a little sound can help ready you to start the day with energy and verve.

Variation:

Instead of moving both hands and feet simultaneously, try stretching the right hand and the left foot away from each other. Then you can switch sides. This gives a nice lengthening across the middle of your body. Explore going back and forth a handful of times.

Benefits:

Stretching like this elongates the spine and stretches many muscles. It's a great wake-up call for the entire body.

Conscious breathing allows you not only to deepen any stretch, but also invigorates the body. Most importantly, starting off your morning by breathing deeply gets you centered for the day ahead.

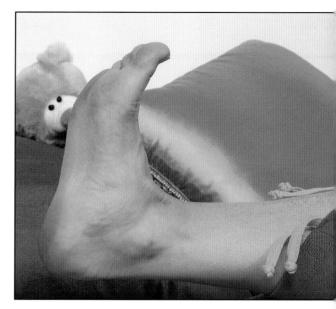

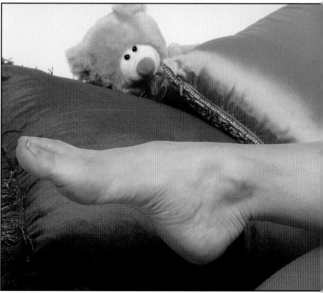

Twist & Sigh

Lying on your back,
Drift your knees to one side.
Let this gentle twist
Unfurl you into the day.

Lying on your back, gently inhale and lift your feet up, bringing the knees a little closer your chest.

Keep your back even on the mattress, as you let the knees fall to one side.

Let your arms fall open in a T-shape. As in all these poses, maybe a sigh will slip from your lips because it feels so good.

Keep the shoulders resting on the mattress, letting your side body gently lengthen and your lower back release. Stay here for a good handful of breaths, then inhale back to center.

Take a moment to readjust, then try the other side. When you finish, release your legs long against the mattress.

Benefits:

Twisting like this unkinks everything,

Lengthens the side body,

Juices up the internal organs,

Brings a feeling of ease, and jump-starts your energy!

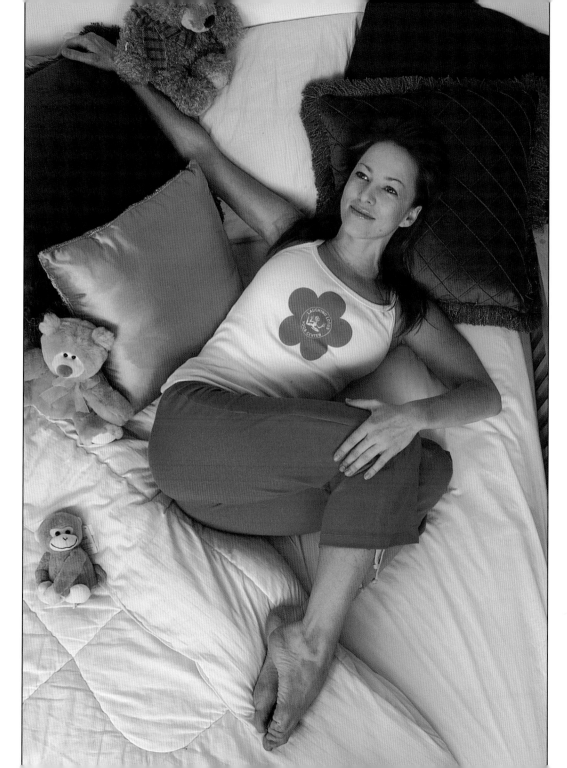

Breakfast Bend

Hug one knee gently into your chest,

Letting your entire back release into the bed.

Open up your feet and ankles.

Follow with a wake-up call for groggy hips.

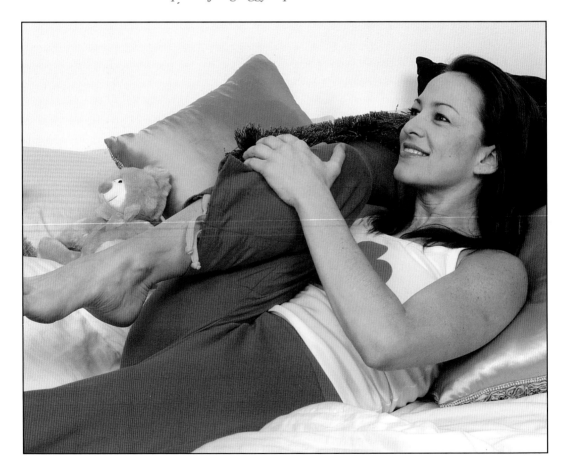

On an inhale, gently lift a knee into your chest. Let your other leg stay long against the mattress.

Hold the shin comfortably with your hands for several breaths, as you explore drawing the knee a little closer towards you.

This is an excellent time to rev up the ankles and feet for the busy day ahead.

Point the toes back and forth as you breath, almost like the foot was waving hello and goodbye. Enjoy stretching the foot smoothly back and forth.

Next, as though the big toe were acting like the minute hand on your alarm clock, trace a nice circle by rotating the ankle clockwise three to five times. Then repeat with a counter-clockwise motion.

To further awaken your lower limbs, try a little "sky-writing."

With your toes, write your name and something amazing you want to celebrate in your near future. Get creative as you prepare your foot for the day's journey ahead.

Variation:

To open up the hips more, you can keep the hands where they are and move the lightly bent leg around in a circle. This circling of the femur (the upper leg bone) opens things up in the hip socket. Keep your motion gentle, remembering your breath, moving almost like you were stirring a magical cauldron nice and slowly. Switch the direction of your movement a few times back and forth. Explore the soft edges of the shape you're making.

Breathing in for one last hug of the knee, you can exhale and release the leg against the bed. After a moment, inhale the other leg to your chest and repeat.

Benefits:

Moving like this opens up the hip and the entire foot and leg.

What a great way to stir things up gently as you awaken. This is a perfect beginning to the day.

Morning Roll

Kneed your knees into yourself.
Butter your lower back against the mattress.
Schmeer yourself from side to side.

Inhale both knees towards the chest. Use your hands to draw them towards yourself gently. Again, make sure this feels comfortable. You want your lower back to release with ease, so avoid all strain.

As a variation, some folks like to cross their ankles with knees spread wide. This can be nice and relaxing for cranky morning hips. See if you prefer that shape more than having your knees together.

Depending on your mood, a little movement can be nice.

You might try subtle circling. You can let your lower back relax into the mattress, while steering the knees around in one direction and then the other.

Another option is a little side-to-side rocking. This can also feel just great.

Benefits:

A morning roll in the hay can be a great way to release your lower back, open the hips, and decompress.

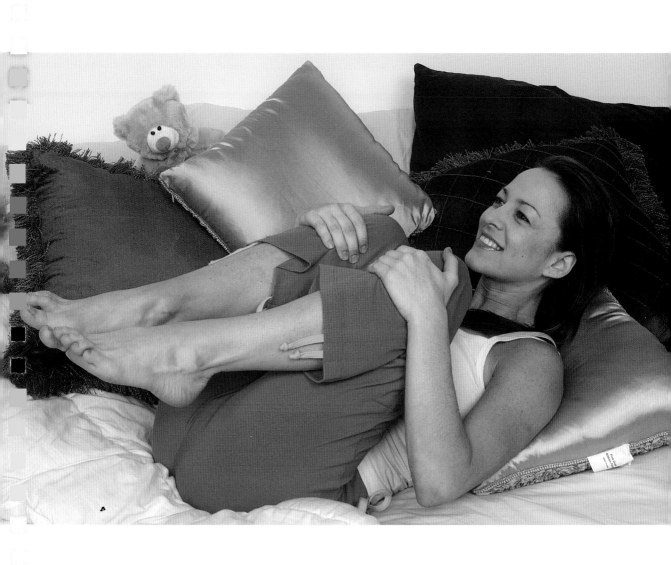

Alarm Clock Rock

Hug yourself affectionately and
Laugh heartily. Then,
Like the kid you are inside—
Rock on up to sit!

Sometimes a little half-somersault action can be quite nice, not only giving yourself a nice back massage, but also letting yourself feel like a kid again. Not a bad way to start the day!

Hug yourself into some version of a little ball, then inhale as you rock forward and exhale as you rock back.

You might enjoy doing this nice and slowly, allowing it to be breath-connecting. Or you could try speeding things up, getting a little "rock and roll" spirit into it. When you're ready, you can rock up to sit comfortably. I think it's fun to let the momentum take you right up into a cross-legged seat if that feels good, but you can always chose to roll to your side and use your hands to sit upright.

Benefits:

Rocking invigorates the body and provides a light massage while toning the belly. Plus hugging yourself gives the back a nice stretch.

And last but not least . . . it's fun!

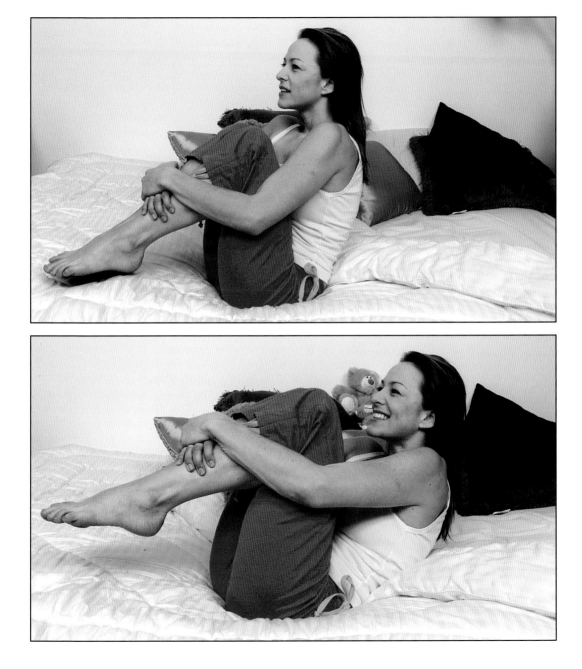

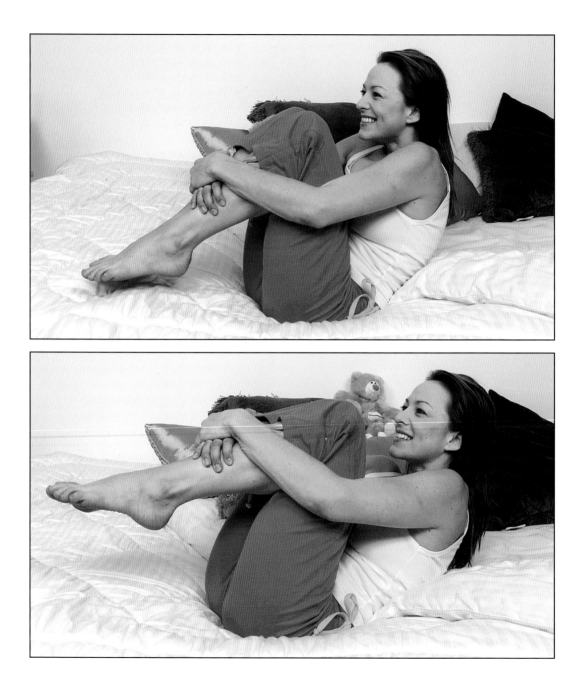

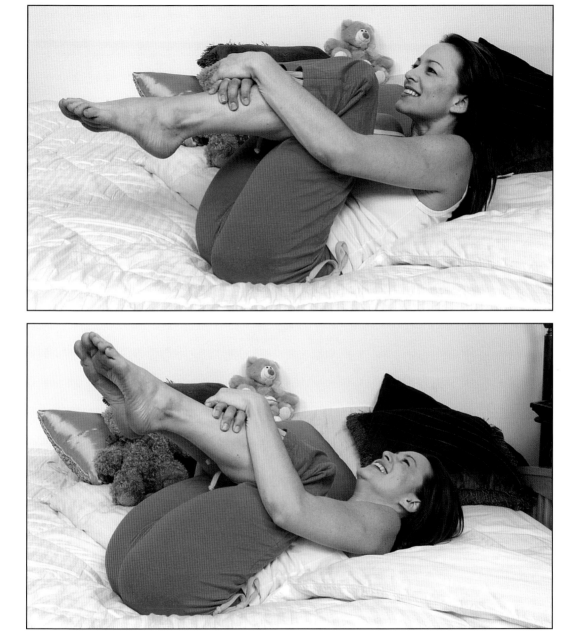

Let Your Head Go

Breathing sweetly,
Drop your head and
Slowly rotate your noggin around.

Rolling around the neck seems pretty simple, but it's good to approach the area respectfully, moving slowly and easily to work through any tightness. Remember: morning stiffness is quite common. That's why *Yoga in Bed* is so important; in the AM you're most in need of loosening up to face the world head-on.

Since you're sitting upright, remember you always have the option of sitting on the edge of several pillows to make yourself more comfortable.

Sometimes it's nice to start with half circles in front. Simply drop your head forward and rotate it around so that the ear approaches the rising shoulder, and then floats back down to explore the other side. After a few times, you might try switching to gentle half-circles in back, making sure not to strain your neck as you slowly move back and forth.

Definitely change direction a few times, letting your movement follow a slow, steady breath.

If you feel any tightness, it might be nice to linger and breathe into that specific area, allowing the tension to be released.

As you do these neck circles, it's a great chance to let any concerns about the world outside your bedroom melt away as well. You might imagine unhelpful, negative thoughts (even any bad dreams!) lightly falling out of your brain, leaving only a positive attitude.

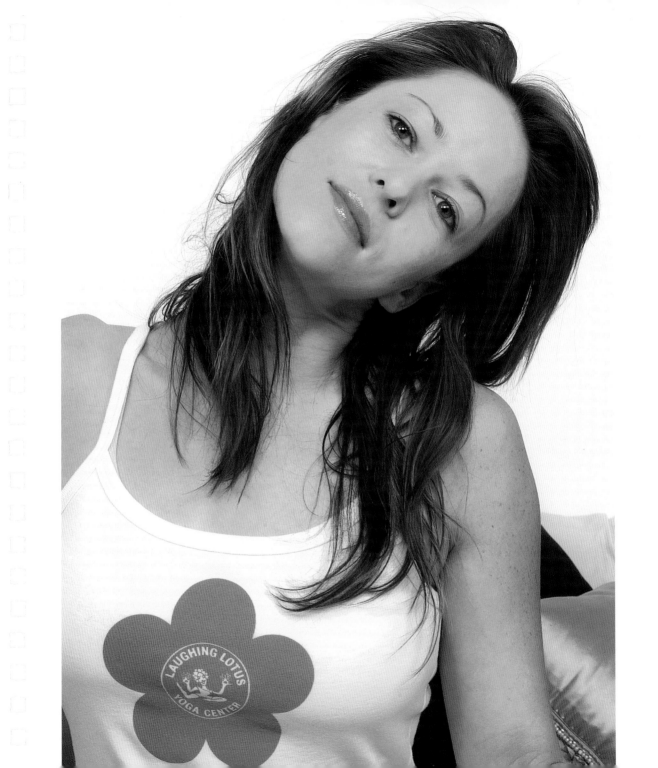

Variation:

For an extra stretch, you can rest one hand over the top of your head, reaching for your opposite ear.

It's good not to use the hand to pull; just allow the soft presence of your hand's extra weight (along with weight of the dropping elbow) to take you deeper into the stretch.

Benefits:

Tension from our daily lives often gets held in the neck. Sudden movements, quirky habits (like cradling a phone between your shoulder and ear), and even sleeping "funny" can result in increased stiffness. A few gentle stretches will help release your neck back to its long, stress-free state.

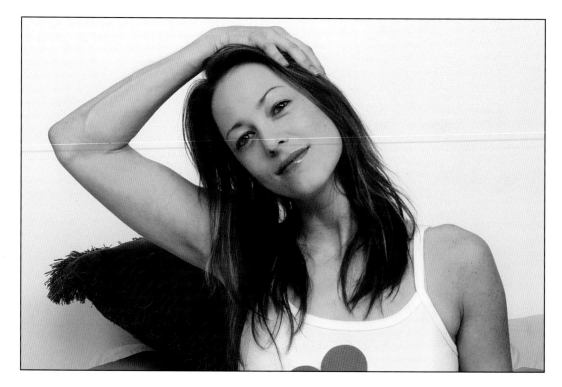

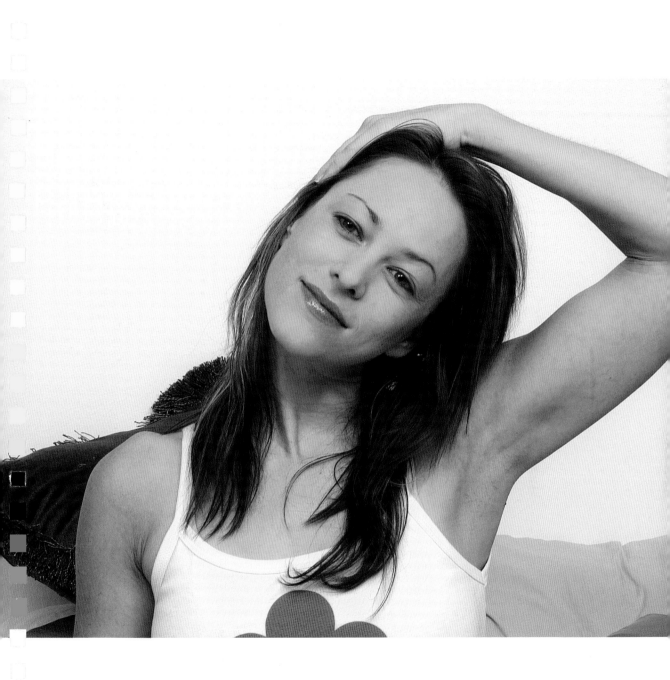

Accepting the Unknown

Yes, No, Maybe.

Practice accepting the Mysteries of Life,

Without leaving your bed.

Sit however you're most comfortable.

Inhale your shoulders up by your ears.

Exhale and gently release them down, letting them drop and back and relax.

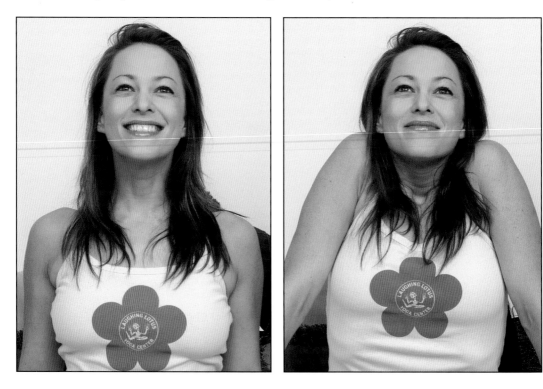

Repeat a few times at this steady, slow pace, moving them up on an inhale, lingering, and then releasing with a slow exhale.

Or, if you want to warm things up, you could pick up the pace of the breath, coordinating it with the up and down of the shoulders. As long as your shoulders are enjoying it, things can speed up and get a little fiery.

There's no need to go faster, however. Many of the most advanced yogis in the world pride themselves on a steady, super slow practice. What's important is how you're feeling in any shape or movement.

Benefits:

Besides warming up and loosening any stiffness in the shoulders, learning to let go can help one's attitude as well.

Sometimes in life the best attitude is admitting you haven't a clue, but are open to whatever life offers. Try to let these shoulder-awakening moves revive your capacity to walk through life with open heart and mind.

Shoulder Circles

Round your shoulders one way,
And then the next,
Releasing them
As you open up your heart.

Life tends to make all of us round our shoulders forward, closing off our heart energy. Yoga works to re-open you, both physically and in your spirit.

Breathing steadily, rotate your shoulders together in an easy, circular direction. Try going up and circling them down and back first.

Let yourself connect with the feeling of your heart lifting as you roll your shoulders back, letting all the kinks of daily living fall away.

Repeat this several times and then switch directions, rolling up and forward.

Play around with some back and forth motions, switching when you feel like it, to let all your burdens slip away.

Benefits:

Looser shoulders—and a softer heart!

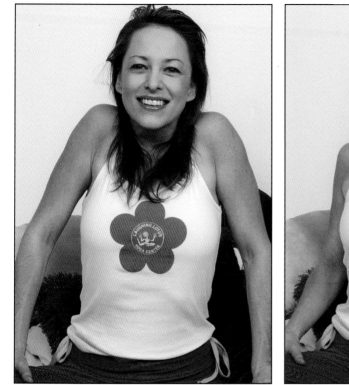
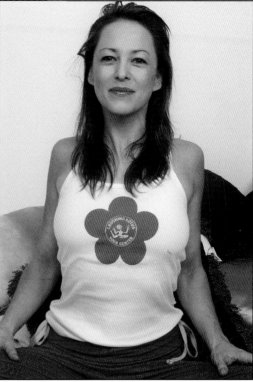

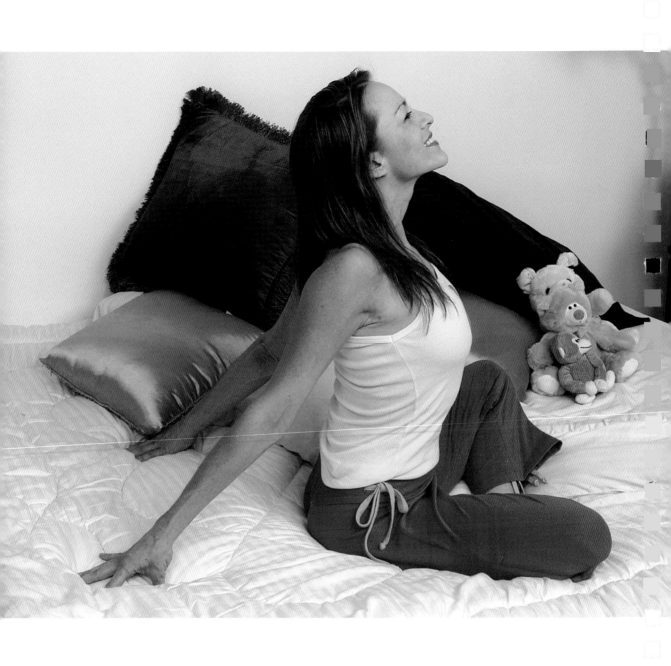

Lift Your Heart

Lift your heart,
Lift your dreams,
Smile into the day ahead.

Sitting any way that's comfortable, walk your hands a little bit behind yourself.

As you inhale, lift your heart up towards the sky, letting your shoulder blades move behind you. Keep your bottom seated, but stretch the chest skyward. Feel your shoulder blades moving closer together on your back. Stay for several breaths if you can. When you return the shape down, exhale, gently releasing the chest.

Repeat several times, allowing the breath to be luxurious and stretchy.

If inspired, feel free to pick up the pace. A single inhalation can elevate your chest and an exhale can let it float down. Only do this if it feels invigorating without being stressful.

Lifting and opening the heart is a fantastic thing to do.

Benefits:

So often life's difficulties make us want to close up, round our shoulders and hide away from the world. It's challenging for everyone to stay open-hearted. Gently expanding the chest like this is the perfect way to face life with a kind heart and a winning attitude.

Wake-Up Spiral

A peaceful twist loosens things up
And starts the day spiraling forward . . . .

Sit comfortably, perhaps in a cross-legged position if that works for you. Any way that's comfortable is fine.

Let your arm reach across in front of you for your opposite knee. Your other hand reaches just behind your back to support you. It might be nice to tent the fingers of the hand in back, keeping the elbows soft. It's good to place the grounding hand towards the center of your back, but only a handful of inches away from you.

Inhale and let your spine grow long and tall. As you exhale, begin to twist in the direction of your back hand.

Don't strain the neck in the twist. Try to have most of the movement come from the belly. It's as though you could bring the navel around to meet the knee you're twisting towards.

Your shoulder also moves into the twist, of course, but again, don't strain anything. Let the navel lead the way.

Stay for a few breaths in the shape, letting yourself twist a little deeper on the exhale, and releasing a little bit out of the twist on the inhale. See if by going in and out of the twist very, very slightly, you end up gently opening deeper into it.

After a moment, inhale as you come back to center. Then journey over to the other side, and repeat.

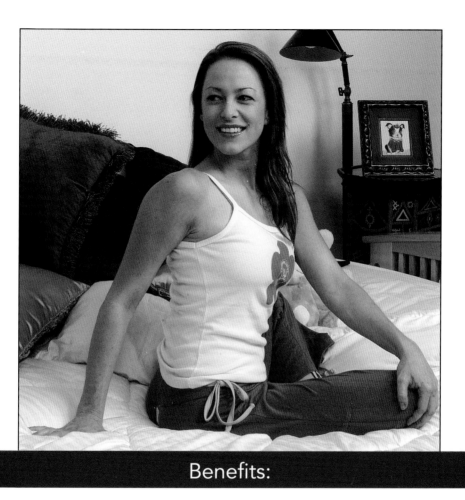

Benefits:

A twist such as this opens and lengthens the spine, releasing tension while toning the belly.

And practicing a twist in this easy way—breathing in and out of the shape—reminds us not to be too fixed in our ideas and approaches. Adding kindness and a little flexibility to our attitude often helps us accomplish more than a hard-driven, relentless approach.

What a perfect reminder of how to approach the challenging people and situations we encounter throughout our day!

Easing into the Day

Sit comfortably with your legs crossed.
Inhale yourself as tall as you can.
Exhale, and ease forward into your future.

As always, be comfortable as you stretch.

One great way to do this is to place a few pillows underneath the back edge of your bottom—this can really help tight hips release a bit.

Before moving forward, it's nice to enjoy a few breaths, letting the inhale in particular help you to sit up tall and stretch your spine.

Then, as you exhale, walk your hands and torso forward. It should feel like you're taking a gentle walk in front of yourself, lengthening out, allowing your heart to release forward and down towards the mattress below.

Of course go only as far as you can comfortably move. Let the entire action be gentle. There's no need to worry about how low you descend; wherever you are is fine.

Spend a few breaths in the shape, perhaps letting a nice full breath lift you up a tiny bit on the inhale, only to have the exhale allow you to release further down and forward.

Another way to make the journey more pleasant is to stack up some blankets or pillows in your lap, or underneath your head. Especially if your hamstrings or lower back are tight, use pillows as shown on the following page. This makes the pose more restful in feeling, allowing you to relax into the padding, rather than feeling any strain from hovering in the air.

I strongly encourage using pillows or blankets whenever there's any strain. In yoga, there's no merit in doing something that feels wrong or is too intense. Try to keep each stretch a little challenging, but easy and soft enough that you can open into it and linger there.

This attitude is so different from many exercise regimes that push you to try harder, that it might take some practice learning to be easy on yourself. (And remember to go easy on yourself about going easy on yourself!)

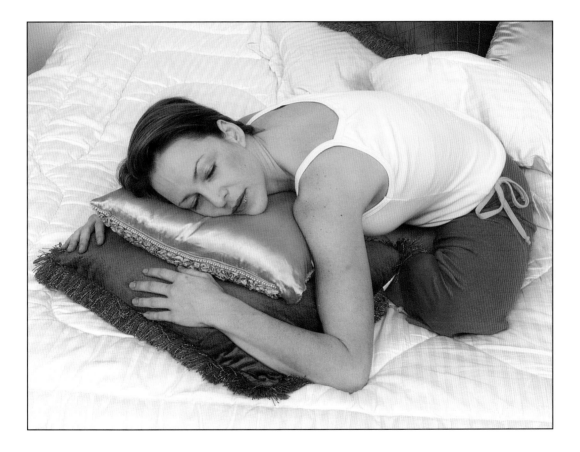

Variation 1:

If you feel comfortable coming forward, you could move into a gentle twist in the forward bend. Walk the hands over to the direction of one knee, keeping the shape low as you twist gently to the side. Let the hands take you out to the side as much as is comfortable, lengthening yourself and weighing down the opposite hip. Spend a few breaths there and then walk back through center. Pay a similar visit to the other side and then return.

Variation 2:

Spread the legs into a wide straddle, being careful not to knock your pet or your favorite stuffed animal out of bed. Inhale tall and again ease forward, enjoying the additional stretch in the hamstrings this pose provides.

This shape can be more challenging for most people—it is for me!—so you might enjoy a little bending of the knees. As always in these sitting positions, a few pillows under the bottom can help release the hips and make the experience friendlier. Or a handful of pillows in front of your torso as you lengthen out might be just the thing.

Or, in all honesty, if this stretch just isn't for you . . . lose it! There are plenty of others that can do the trick. The last thing anyone needs is for their yoga to stress them out!

Benefits:

Sitting cross-legged helps open up the hips.

Stretching forward, hamstrings receive a wake-up call.

Forward bending stretches the spine and strengthens the muscles of the back.

Especially with a bunch of pillows, there's a terrific possibility of letting yourself melt as you move forward. Once the straining is gone, there's a tremendous potential to just let go—and that's what yoga's all about!

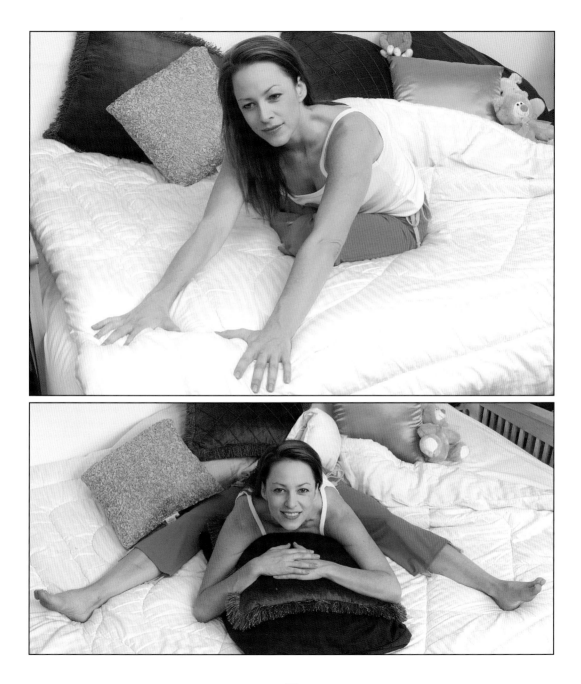

I'm A Little Tea Pot Stretch

Sit comfortably.
Inhale and raise your arm skyward.
Exhale, stretching into the great day ahead.

Sit comfortably and allow yourself to be lifted tall in your spine.

Breathe in as you raise your arm towards the sky. As you exhale, you can bring your other arm by your side on the bed to gently support you. Keep lifting the lifted arm, palm facing down and let yourself tilt towards the arm on the ground.

Try to keep both sides of your hips weighted down equally so that you feel the stretch from the side of your hip through the fingertips. In other words, don't get carried away and lean too much into the lifting arm's direction. Stay anchored in your seat. You'll get much more stretch that way.

Remember to keep the neck long and relaxed as you look up. Soften the neck rather than extending it too far into the stretch.

Encourage a little turning of the chest skyward as you lift your heart towards the ceiling.

As the arm reaches away, keep your shoulders comfortably resting on the back. Feel that you can bring the upper arm and the ear closer together as you lengthen the side of your body.

Linger in the pose for several breaths, perhaps sinking a little deeper into the stretch on an exhale, then lifting a bit out of the shape on an inhale. A handful of breaths on each side should feel absolutely terrific.

Windmill Variation:

After you've warmed yourself up, if you'd like a little more excitement, you might try switching side to side with each breath. Simply inhale, then exhale to the right side. Inhale back up to straight and center, then exhale to the left. Try this a few times without rushing. Keep the movement nice and slow and deeply connected to the breath.

Benefits:

Stretching this way lengthens the side body and opens the chest and shoulders. Moving in two directions also helps tone the tummy.

Finally, moving back and forth reminds us that there are always two sides to everything!

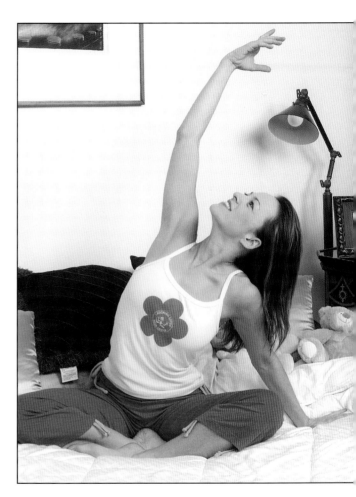

Morning Juicer

Twirling around,
The hips start to open,
The shoulders get lose,
And your energy starts to rise.

Sitting comfortably and cross-legged, bring your hands to your knees, keeping your elbows bent and soft.

Inhale and let your torso lean forward, letting your elbows point out to the side and steer you around. Move in a circle, exhaling as you spiral back and inhaling when you come forward.

There are no rules here. Just let yourself loosen up, breathing into the circling shapes you're making. Reverse directions a few times. Or stay in the front for a while, then linger with half circles in the back. What's important is that you're finding the way to best open yourself up. Be adventurous yet gentle as you explore.

Feel free to be playful in the looseness. Let yourself laugh aloud if you tip in one direction or another. Don't worry—you're safe in bed.

Benefits:

Circling opens the hips and laughter opens the soul.

"Getting a little tipsy" like this is a great way to start the day!

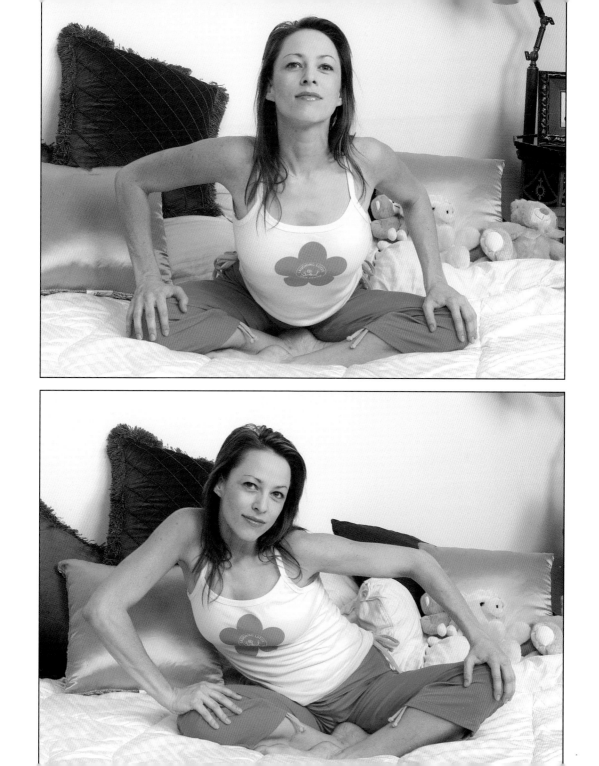

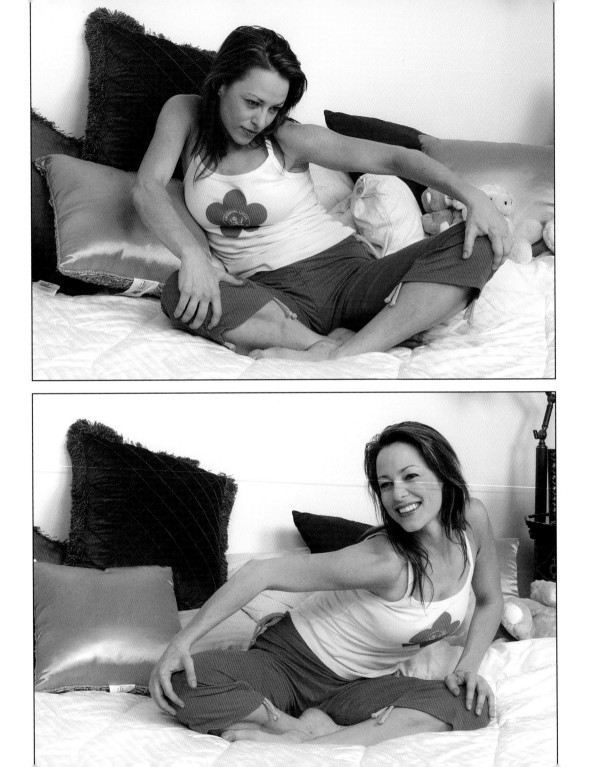

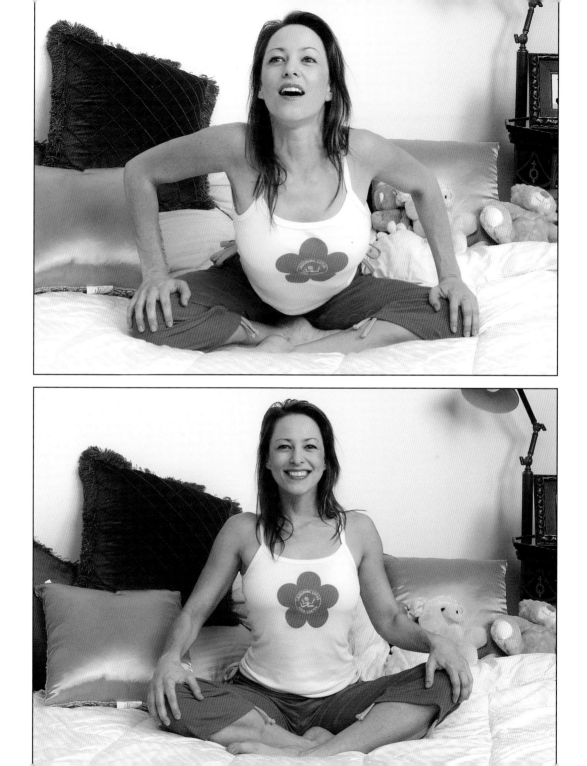

Sun Celebration

Inhale and raise your arms to greet the day.
Exhale, feeling centered and grounded.

Sit however is comfortable for you. Let your hands drop naturally to your sides.

Breathe in deeply and lift your open palms skyward so that they meet either in prayer above your head or simply stay wide and uplifted. You can linger here for a few breaths, letting your shoulder blades soften down away from your ears, but also letting your heart be lifted.

Exhale slowly, lowering your arms, palms facing down, to land by your sides. Continue inhaling as you move your arms up and exhaling on the way down.

It's nice to keep a little life in the hands as you move them. The fingers might be spread or together, but feel a sense of the hands connecting with the breath as you move in each direction.

Let the exalted feeling of raising your arms lift up your spirit.

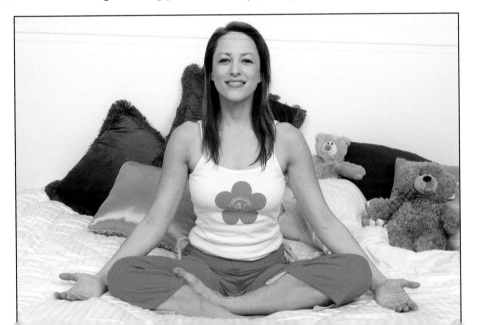

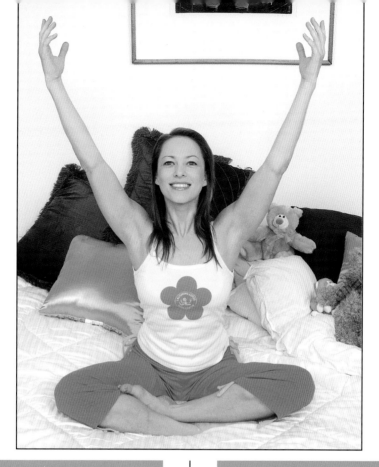

Variation:

If you'd like to move a little faster and warm the body, you could inhale the hands up and exhale them down, moving directly on each breath. Enjoy a few rounds as you salute the rising sun and everything that's ahead for your day.

Benefits:

Moving like this opens the shoulders and chest, improving breathing and circulation as it invigorates the body.

And opening your hands and heart upward with the breath can be a wonderful way to express devotion to whatever it is that you find sacred and special in your life.

Rising Lion

Learn to laugh at yourself.
Make your funniest face
And growl!

Yup, this is really a yoga pose. It's called *Simhasana* in Sanskrit.

Inhale, then exhale, sticking the tongue towards the chin and crossing your eyes. Roar!

Benefits:

The pose obviously stretches the muscles of the face, and lets you express whatever crazy noises you feel like making.

Most importantly, it lets you not take yourself so seriously.

We yogis can take things in stride because we're able to laugh at our experiences.

What a terrific way to start the day: making a funny face and roaring out loud with crazy, child-like joy!

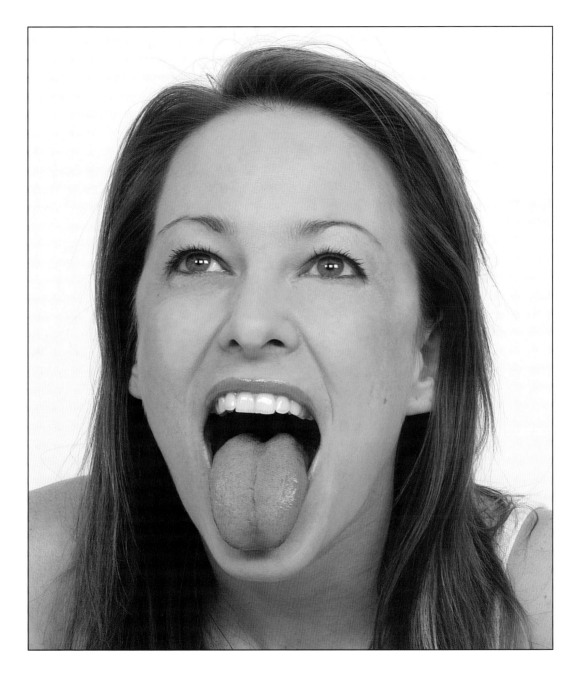

Breath of Fire

Inflame your breath with passion
To fire up your day.

Breathing in and out means you're alive.

Breathing in and out deeply and slowly means you're practicing yoga and living a richer, fuller, and ultimately calmer life.

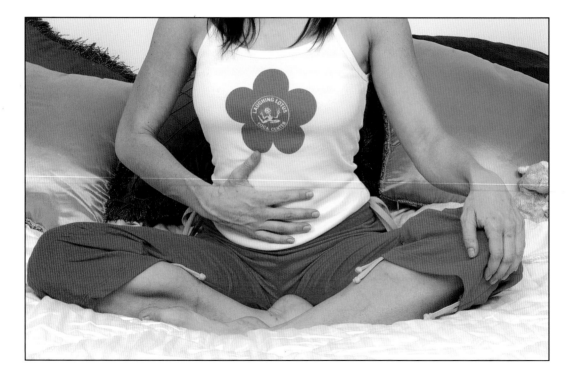

But there are also yoga breaths designed to be invigorating and enlivening. One of these is Breath of Fire.

The breath is still through the nose, except it's very fast and fluttery.

First, find your favorite comfortable seated position. Make sure your shoulder blades are nestled on your back and that your heart is open and lifted. Take a few normal breaths to center yourself.

Then approach Breath of Fire this way: open your mouth and for a few seconds pant like a dog. Then close your mouth and keep that same, energetic feeling while breathing rapidly in and out through the nose. Try to keep the breath light though, with a fluttery attitude. You want nothing to be forced, just a steady, pulse-like feeling. You can rest your hand on your belly to feel the light, rapid movement of your breath.

This breath is highly invigorating. Enjoy it for however long you can without getting winded. Perhaps you can work your way up to thirty seconds, a minute, even two or more.

After a round of Breath of Fire, it's nice to close your eyes and breathe in and out deeply again, savoring the energy you've generated. If you like, a second round might be interesting.

When you're finished, keep your eyes closed and spend a few minutes contemplating the equally exciting day ahead.

Benefits:

Wonderfully invigorating for the entire system, particularly strengthening the abdomen and all the other muscles used in breathing.

A little getting fiery with your breath can help you stay passionate about your life.

Coffee Cup Meditation

Start your day right . . .
Celebrate all the great joys in your life,
Looking forward to more ahead.

Meditation doesn't have to be done for hours in a cave, or on a beach watching the sunset, or even in an ashram, temple, or church.

Indeed, some meditations are about "emptying" the mind and trying to "stop thinking." If that instruction works for you, that's terrific. Personally, I find a meditation with a focus much easier in the beginning then trying to empty my mind.

Why not begin every day the way you like best: with a steaming cup of coffee or tea—or a delicious fruit smoothie if that's for you? But as a yogi, combine your caffeine or sugar rush with a jolt of thankfulness.

First, feel the corners of your mouth gently rise. Simply bringing an easy smile to your face begins to soften a worried brain.

Second, let your mind come back to your breath. Easy in and out through the nose, letting that be a calming focus as you inhale those delicious java aromas.

Third, focus on your coffee. It's a universal truth that what you focus on expands; I try to focus on the positive. Therefore, I suggest spending a few moments each

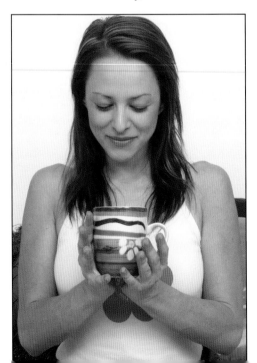

morning lost in the delights of your coffee, counting your many blessings and soaking in gratitude.

Allow all your attention to stay in the present moment, savoring the smell, the warmth, and the taste of a delicious latte, cappuccino, or house blend.

All your thoughts regarding your to-do list and the fuss waiting for you at work, or getting the kids ready, or whatever real world stresses you face can wait for five minutes while you just savor your breath— or that delicious sip of java.

Indulge yourself by *not* indulging all the cares and concerns that cry out for your attention. For a few minutes, simply savor the moment, letting your mind settle on the simple pleasures of your breath and your morning brew.

Sip by sip, you'll set the perfect tone for the rest of your day.

If a beverage isn't the thing that turns you on, select something else: maybe a picture of your family or your favorite pet. An image of a hero or role model who inspires you. Or some symbol of a concept, goal, or ideal that you're striving towards.

It doesn't matter what you choose, so much as that you allow yourself to truly focus on something inspiring, letting everything else fade away for a few minutes. You'll feel centered and uplifted.

Starting out with such a strong morning moment will give you a spiritual "home base" to return to whenever challenges in the day arise. By making the firm decision to be positive and have a great day, you've already taken the biggest step to making that a reality.

Benefits

Smiling relaxes (and prevents) frown lines.

Slowing down the rushing flow of thoughts eases stress.

A centered, grateful moment is the best foundation for your day.

Savoring the present is the secret to lasting happiness.

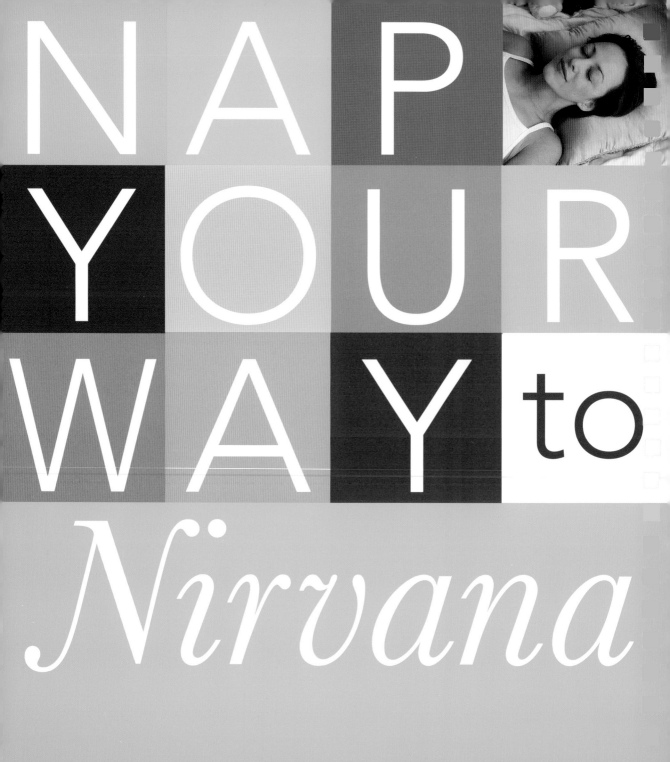

NAP YOUR WAY to Nirvana

What do Salvador Dali, Thomas Edison, Napoleon, Winston Churchill, Albert Einstein, John F. Kennedy, and Bill Clinton have in common? All of these men are among history's many famous nappers. Think about it: these men were often running countries and empires, yet they recognized the need to stop themselves and get the rest they needed. Winston Churchill was particularly adamant about the benefits of a noonday snooze:

You must sleep sometime between lunch and dinner, and no halfway measures. Take off your clothes and get into bed. That's what I always do. Don't think you will be doing less work because you sleep during the day. That's a foolish notion held by people who have no imagination. You will be able to accomplish more. You get two days in one— well, at least one and a half, I'm sure. When the war started, I had to sleep during the day because that was the only way I could cope with my responsibilities.

—Winston Churchill

They were not only successful innovators and leaders in their respective realms, they were even proud of their creativity in their pursuit of ZZZs. For example, Salvador Dali would let himself drift off in a chair, holding an object in his hand over a metal bowl. When he moved into deep sleep, his hand would release and the clanking noise would awaken him.

Many studies agree that a short rest can be extremely reviving during the middle of the day. Evidence exists to demonstrate that a mid-afternoon nap can improve work performance and elevate mood. My personal experience confirms this. A short mid-day snooze is often the perfect answer whenever I feel my energy ebbing.

While many cultures—particularly the Spanish—support the noonday siesta, employers may not be supportive of workers taking a sleep break. This is changing, however, and you can always present your boss with information from The National Sleep Foundation and other sources confirming the greater efficiency and numerous health benefits naps offer his or her hard-workers. And, best thing of all, napping's a corporate perk that costs the employer nothing whatsoever!

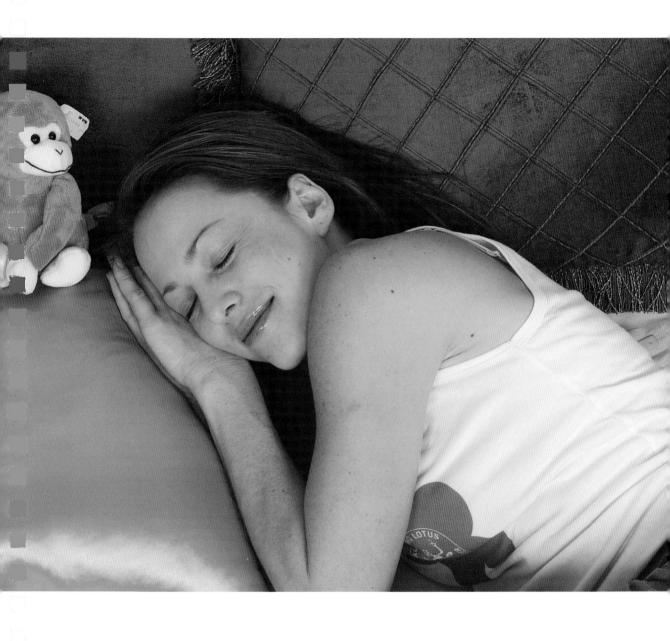

Tips For Power Napping

It seems like it would be quite simple to just curl up and nod off, but a little knowledge and planning can maximize your naptime dosing. Here are the essentials:

Commit to the right amount of time

It's difficult to contradict Churchill, but most studies show that the 20–30 minutes is the best amount of time for a nap. There's some research supporting Churchill's belief that the 1.5 hour schedule is best, but that's often difficult for most folks to budget into their busy day. (If you can, however, how fantastic to treat yourself so well!)

In general, researchers feel that the time between 30 minutes and an hour and a half places one in the middle of a different sleep cycle. When that's interrupted, it results in a groggy feeling. No one wants to nap only to wake up feeling even more tired.

Best advice: experiment a bit with the right sleep time for you, knowing that more isn't necessarily better.

Schedule it in

Planning your nap routine will help reinforce the importance of good sleep in your life. If you schedule your afternoon to factor in your nap, it's much more likely to happen than if it's seized between the cracks of your appointments.

Psychologically, it also helps to know that you have a break scheduled. It can help your attitude and energy, before, during, and after your shut-eye.

Use an alarm clock

It's good to have an alarm clock and set it so that your nap doesn't go astray. The nap is designed to improve your efficiency and productivity. The last thing you want is to sleep the afternoon away!

And, as per the research cited above, you want to make sure you sleep within the right sleep cycles so that you wake up refreshed . . . not craving more sleep.

Set yourself up

Many people take nap breaks in their cars or at their desks. You may have limitations on the how, where, and when you take your nap, but try to make yourself as comfortable as possible. A pillow or a blanket can really make the experience nicer, and will help you drift off more quickly to maximize your shuteye minutes.

Practicing letting go

Flashback to kindergarten. Recall your naptime successes.

No matter how mammoth the responsibilities of life get—even if you're not Churchill or JFK—realize that you, too deserve that little bit of afternoon delight in your day.

And best of all, this letting go is in itself close to the very heart of yoga: a true calming of the storms of the mind.

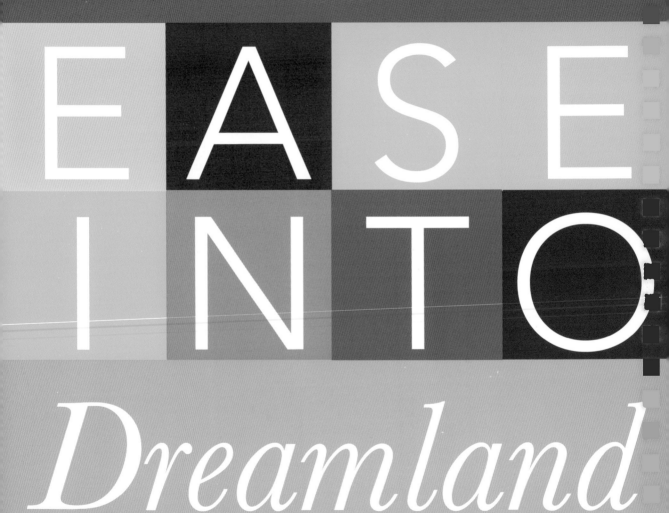

Evening Poses:

EASE INTO

Dreamland

Shifting into Sleep Mode

The poses in this section of *Yoga in Bed* are perfect for unwinding at the end of a long day. For the soundest sleep, start unwinding early in the evening—long before you get into your pajamas—rather than right before turning out the lights. If you've come in from a late night at the office or have just put the kids to bed, for instance, give yourself some time to do a relaxed, mellow activity like these postures before segueing directly into your sleep.

If you watch television before bed each night, it might be good to shut the set off fifteen minutes to a half-hour before going to bed. Let your brain have some time without the added stimulation. Even if television helps you relax after a hard day, it still demands your attention and provides a lot of distracting, noisy stimulation. Shutting it off for those fifteen to thirty minutes before you're ready to sleep lets your brain "cool off" completely. In this information-on-demand age, we sometimes forget that we can't just flip the switch and change the channel with ourselves as easily as we can with a remote.

For the same reason, don't exercise vigorously too close to bedtime. You don't want to rev up your metabolism and over-stimulate yourself. Budget enough time between your "gym" work out and *Yoga in Bed* stretches in order to smoothly downshift your gears. Also consider establishing a simple sleep ritual such as a hot bath or a cup of non-caffeinated tea each night before retiring, to cue your body and mind into sleep mode.

This next set of poses will help to do the same:

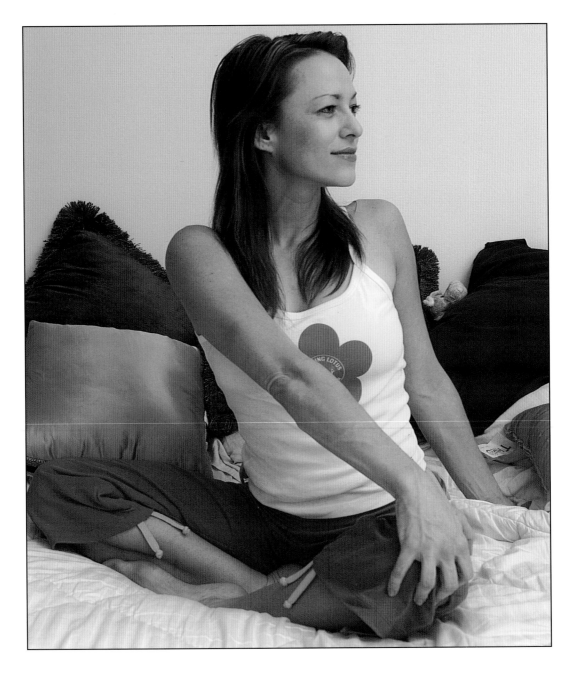

Winding Down Twist

At the end of the day,
Twist away your stress
To find sweet release.

This morning twist is also excellent before retiring.

No matter how much yoga you practice, there are going to be challenges all along the way. Winding down before bed with a deep, soothing twist, lets the day's accumulated tensions melt away.

As before, reach across yourself with one arm, the other hand behind your back steadying you. Fingers can be nicely tented in the back hand, so you have lots of height in the shape.

Inhale and lengthen your spine. Exhale and twist.

Keep this sweet rhythm over several breaths in and out.

Remember: keep the neck relaxed. Moving from the belly lets the twist come from the right place. Enjoy, inhale as you return to center, and then try the other side.

Benefits:

Twists can be very releasing, so make sure you linger for a handful of breaths on each side. The feeling should be that you're gently wringing away any stress that's gotten lodged in your spine, cleansing yourself of any residual tension from the day.

Afterward, you should feel as though by gently twisting you've somehow rinsed the spine clean, with your mind therefore feeling much calmer, too.

Relax and Restore _____

The next four poses—CHILD'S POSE, FLOATING TO DREAMLAND, NIGHTTIME GODDESS STRETCH, and UPSIDE DOWN RELAXATION—are all terrific ways to restore and relax yourself at the end of the day. They allow the body to open gently, stretching and lengthening you even as they soothe you. They are great before bed.

There's never a need to rush in yoga, and that's doubly so when practicing these kind of laid-back, hang out poses. If one's feeling particularly great, why not stick with it? A few minutes—as long as there's no strain—can be completely delightful. Once you're experienced in the pose, you can VERY gradually enjoy staying a little longer each time you practice. So while you might sample all of them or any combination on different nights, feel free to pick one or two that feel right to linger in longer. Trust your ability to sense what your body needs and how you feel while staying in the pose.

Always remember that you're the best judge if the pose is working for you. Be intuitive and keep "checking in" with how you're feeling. These poses are all so great, however, that I really think with the right blankets and pillows, you'll have an incredibly restful time.

Child's Pose

Perfected by babies and children everywhere,
Breath deep into this pose,
The perfect prelude to sleep.

Some folks find that a forward bend from kneeling is more comfortable than sitting.

Let your knees be wide enough apart to allow a stack of pillows (or a rolled up blanket) to come in front of you. The feet don't need to touch, but let the tops of your feet be flat on the mattress. You don't want to have a torqued feeling of the feet twisting too much.

If you experience any discomfort in your knees, ankles, or feet, place a small pillow (or a towel) right at the bend at the back of the knee. It should help.

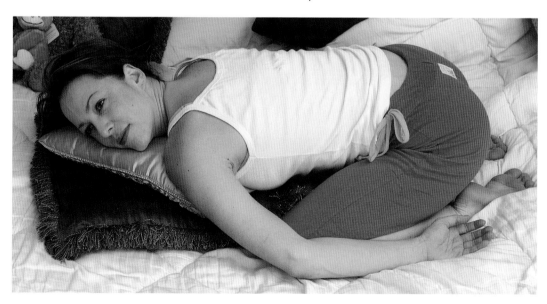

Leaning forward, sit back on your heels. Your bottom might not get all the way down and that's OK. Just enjoy lengthening in that direction while letting yourself melt down and forward.

Like all yoga poses, there are lots of variations possible here, based on what feels like a comfortable stretch.

For example, your hands might reach forward. Or you might find you enjoy letting the arms drift back towards the feet. Wherever you place your hands and arms, make sure it's the most relaxing choice.

Some folks prefer face down into the pillows, while others bring the head to one side. Alternate your head to the other side after a while, particularly if there's any strain in the neck.

Most importantly, let your mind close up shop. Really allow yourself to feel the childlike sense of letting go this pose can bring.

Benefits:

The back releases. Shoulders melt. Feelings of childlike ease and freedom lead the body toward surrender.

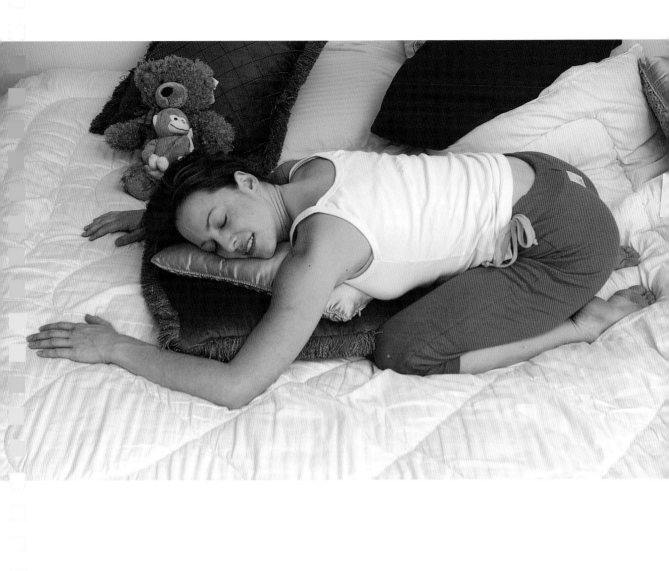

Floating Off to Dreamland

Floating off to dreamland,
Release your heart and mind,
Letting your breath flow like water.

Pillows and padding make this a splendid, deeply relaxing opening. Experiment with stacking pillows and blankets, until you find the most pleasing placement.

Sit with a bunch of pillows and blankets by your side. One pillow (or bunch of pillows) will go directly underneath your shoulder blades. This will lift and allow your chest to open.

Another small pillow underneath your neck can also feel great.

Finally, many people feel that a rolled-up blanket or a few pillows for underneath your knees can help make the pose more relaxing for the lower back.

(One more "pillow plug:" eye pillows that cover the eyes can be extremely soothing right before sleep. They're often scented with lavender or other herbs, to help signal your brain to turn on its "snooze" setting.)

As you lie back on top of your padding, take the time to adjust the heights of blankets and pillows so that everything feels great.

There should be enough of a lift in the chest that you feel some letting go, but not so much that anything feels strained. As always, padding under the knees can help the lower back.

After you make yourself comfy-cozy, simply let go. Let the blankets, pillows, and gravity do all the work. Breathe and sink into the shape, enjoying every minute of it.

Relax and Restore

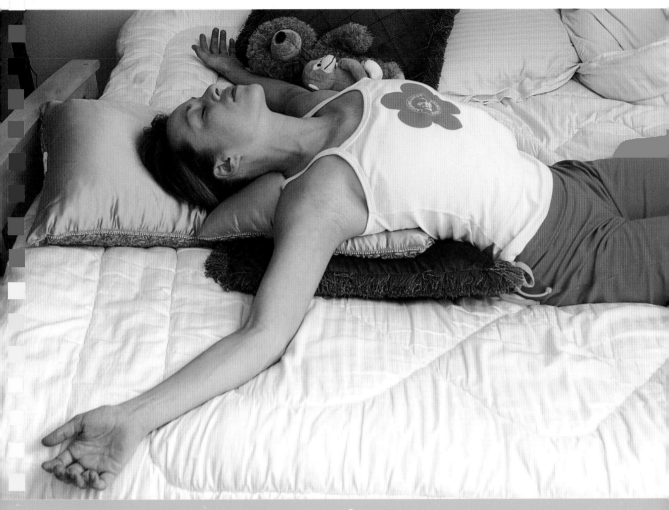

Benefits:

Enjoy your spine moving into a sweet, rippling shape. The heart is being opened and a backbend is being sustained, but with minimal effort.

The breath, too, flows like water. The entire pose makes you want to sigh and enjoy the blissful breath.

Nighttime Goddess Stretch
(Good for the guys too!)

Easy does it.
Everything melts.
Let gravity do the work to
Open your hips and your heart!

Go crazy with pillows, especially you guys who are tight in the hips and find this pose challenging. Even if you are flexible here, take the time you need to set yourself up right, so this pose can work its restorative wonders.

Approach it lying down with pillows in ready reach.

Bring the soles of your feet together and draw them close to your groin, allowing your knees to drift apart.

Place pillows underneath the thighs as they drift down and away, knees diamonding out to the sides.

You might enjoy another small pillow under your head so your neck stays long.

Several pillows or a rolled up blanket might be nice right underneath your shoulder blades.

Lift up your pelvis for a moment the tiniest bit away from the mattress. While you're hovering, curl your lower back flat, dipping the tailbone—that last bit of bone in your spine—down towards your feet.

Then you can lower yourself down to the mattress, once again releasing yourself and letting go.

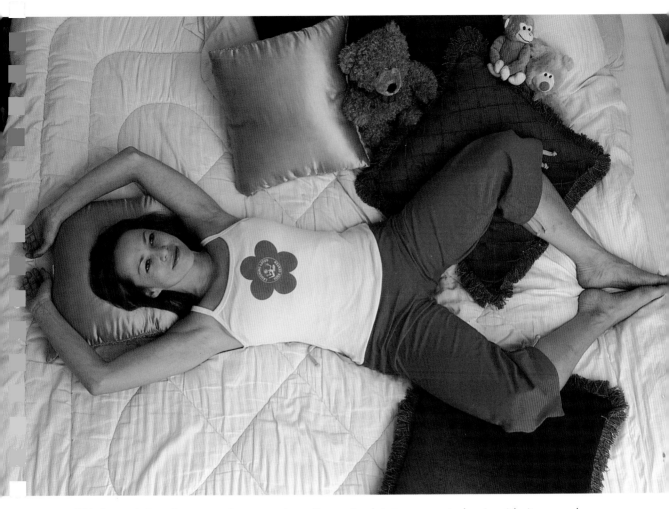

This is a subtle adjustment, but sometimes if your back is too curvy to begin with, it can make a difference. What's essential is that everything should feel quite sweetly released.

Besides the pillows under each thigh, you can always butterfly the knees up an inch or two and then re-release them. This movement can be quite subtle, but it prevents a feeling of too much intensity in the groin if that starts to occur.

Let your arms drift above your head, allowing your chest to expand. It feels fantastic to take a few easy, deep breaths here. Enjoy how sweet it is to inhale and let the whole torso expand with the fullness of the breath, followed by an easy exhale and a letting go. Delicious . . .

Or you might find that at bedtime, it might be more relaxing to keep the hands loose and out to the sides. The chest is still opening, but this has a calming, less vigorous effect than hands above the head.

Stay for a few breaths. You might enjoy looking up at the ceiling, picturing all the positive things you're grateful for along with what you're striving to create for your future.

Remember, the point of the pillows is to de-stress you. If there's too much tension anywhere— particularly in the groin—then add more pillows or gently come out of the pose.

As always, mind your breath in an easy-going way, allowing yourself to further let go in each and every moment.

Note: Sometimes this pose might be a little stressful for tight hips and groins, so go easy and move out of it gently. It helps create a powerful, deep opening, so in the beginning be sensitive to any discomfort. You can work up over time to a few minutes or more.

To come out of the pose, let the hands frame the underneath sides of the thighs, as you draw the knees back together. Extend the legs long to stretch everything in the other direction.

Benefits:

Hips and thighs open.

Pelvis and belly release.

Chest expands with arms lifted.

A feeling of emotional expansion can bloom.

Upside Down Relaxation

Just when you feel
Like climbing up the wall
Throw your legs up one instead!

For this terrific pose you obviously need a headboard or your bed placed against the wall with nothing in the way.

Everyone has a different way of getting into this shape. Here's the way I've found best for myself.

I sit facing the wall, and then I pivot over so that my side is about a foot away the wall.

With my side parallel to the wall, I lie back down, swinging my legs skyward and up the wall. This move is pretty simple but it may take a few tries before you find the right distance to be comfortable. I always adjust, moving my bottom closer or further away, depending on what feels right.

As always in yoga, you have choices about your position. The closer your bottom is to the wall, the more vigorous a hamstring stretch you're going to get. Since we're doing this before bed, you may or may not want that much activity taking place. Especially for an evening restorative pose, you want to make choices that feel conducive to a restful mind/body connection. It's a personal decision. Rather than keeping the legs rigid against the wall, you can always bend the knees a bit.

Make sure you have some pillows and blankets at the ready. Some folks feel that the softness of the mattress is enough for them, but others enjoy a little extra padding to open up the shape a bit more. Experiment and see what you like.

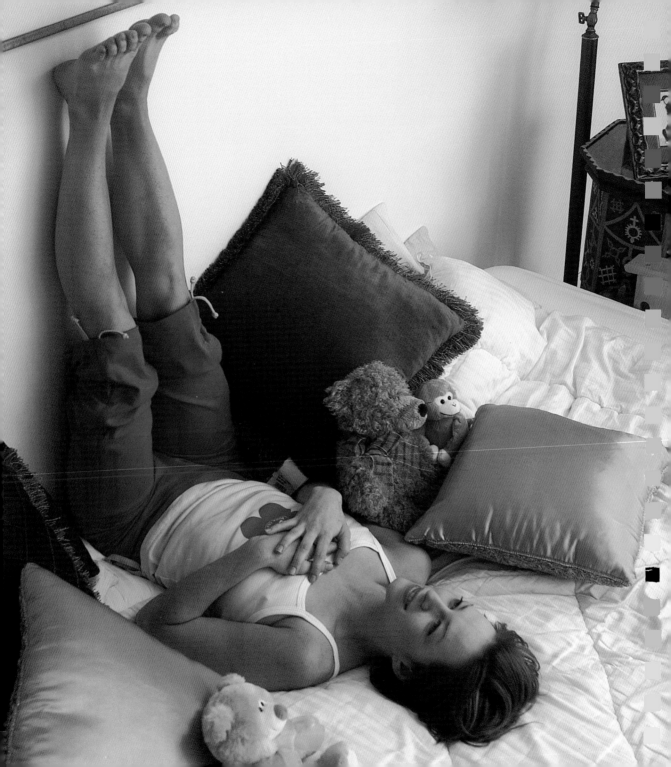

Lift your pelvis slightly and slip the pillows underneath you, so that they fill up the space from wall to waistband. There should be a gently opening feeling in the chest.

Hands can go above your head if you want to open your chest, or by your side if you want a more tranquil feeling. A little pillow can be wonderful underneath the neck as well.

Make sure your chin is relaxed and not moving into your neck forcefully.

This is a terrific pose for anyone, especially if you've had a hard time being on your feet all day. Everything just pools down nicely, as though your cares were spilling gently into a tropical lagoon. Let them wash away as you get ready to drift off to dreamland.

Coming out of the pose may require a little experimenting as you maneuver but is really quite simple. First, lift up your bottom and remove any padding or pillows. Then, keeping the knees and legs bent, you can roll off to the side. Take a few breaths as you relax, and then gently come back up to sit.

Benefits:

A terrific stress reliever, this pose opens up your chest. This means that your heart and lungs are gently refreshed.

In addition, this pose is great for people who spend the day on their feet, or have any swelling in the legs.

There's something terrifically quieting about it as well. Next time you feel like life's "driving you up the wall". . . maybe you should go there—the yoga way!

Bedtime Bending

Let go,
Fold into yourself,
Find the calm within.

This one might be the one to save for last, as it allows you to fold right into yourself. Its soft quality makes it perfect right before sleep time.

At the end of the day, I highly recommend using pillows in the forward bend . . . as many as you want.

Although the idea of forward bending might seem straightforward and simple, this kind of pose can often be extremely challenging for many people. It doesn't seem like it would be difficult to be in a forward bending shape, but it often can be. Pillows can change your relationship to the pose so that it becomes a chance to relax and let go.

Sit in whatever way feels comfortable.

When you bend forward, if there's any stiffness in the spine or hips, fill your lap with a bounty of pillows. Definitely let your head find one as well.

Again, coordinating the breath with the subtle motion of inhaling, feel your lungs lift you a millimeter higher, then exhale and let yourself soften deeper and further forward. Try this a few times, and then abandon all effort. Just let yourself go.

Be sensitive to your needs in the pose. Depending on how far forward you are, you might want additional pillows so that the head isn't strained at all but is supported. Allow yourself to be completely comfortable in the shape.

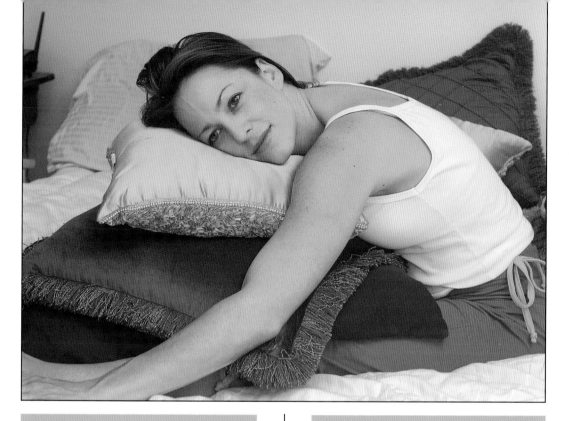

Variation:

If it feels comfortable, sitting up you might straighten both your legs. Then fill up the space in front of you with as many pillows as you want. Make sure the head can be released into the sweet hill of pillows in front of you. Don't care how forward your hands reach—there's no prize for reaching your toes or anywhere else in yoga. Just breathe deep and let go.

Benefits:

A forward bend like this lengthens the spine, stretches the hamstrings, loosens the hips. Done with pillows and without strain, it also quiets the brain, allowing you a few introspective moments as you draw into yourself.

What perfect preparation for sleep!

Clearing Your Mind:
3 Simple Practices

Rub the Slate Clean

Rub the slate clean to
Free your mind.

With your right open palm, for a few breaths gently rub the space between your brows—called the third eye—using the heel of the palm of your hand. Imagine that all the worries of your day are falling by the wayside.

Without irritating your skin, generate a little heat. Then, when the feeling's right, enjoy a deep inhale. As you exhale the palm slowly floats away from your smiling face. Know you've wiped the slate clean.

Benefits:

Combining the movement and energy of the hand with the intention of releasing negativity, doubles the effectiveness of this practice of letting go.

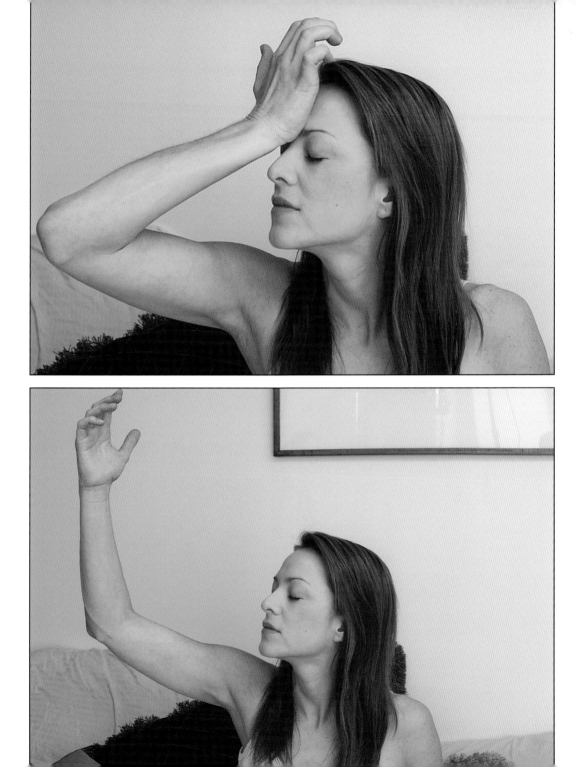

Massage Your Mind

Wash the day's residue away,
As easily as you wash your hair.

Starting at the hairline, run your fingers through your hair, gently massaging your scalp. Let them roam over your entire head, playfully letting them drift through your hair and over your ears.

Self-massage feels terrific, and once again, as you breathe in and out deeply and with ease, you can practically feel all your cares melting away.

Benefits:

Just another wonderful technique for the constant yoga practice of letting go!

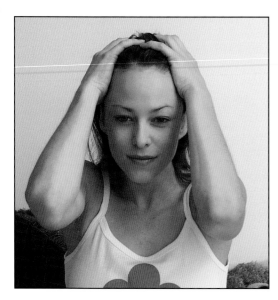
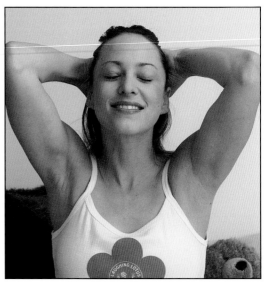

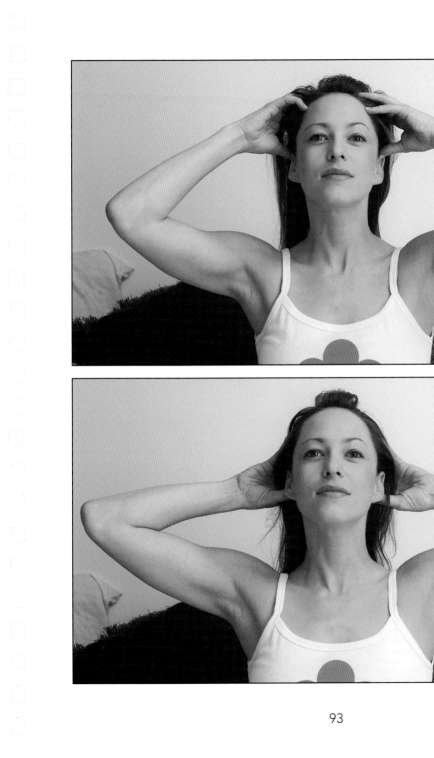

Blissful Breath

Enjoy alternative breathing
As a soothing exploration of yourself.

Nothing evens out the mind like alternate nostril breathing.

Try this sitting or lying down. You might even enjoy it in one of the previous restorative poses.

This breath is a fantastic way to de-stress and center anytime, taking only a few minutes to produce a deeply calming effect.

You'll use your right hand to switch back and forth between nostrils. Curl your first and second fingers in, leaving your thumb and fourth finger to do the work. This is the traditional shape of the hand—hand poses are called *mudras*—but honestly anything that works will be fine.

Your right hand floats in front of your nose. Your thumb gently blocks your right nostril, as you inhale through the left. Pause for a second, and release the thumb and let the fourth finger (or any finger that's available) block the left nostril to exhale. Empty out completely on the right, then inhale on the same side.

You'll get the rhythm pretty soon. After each exhale, inhale on the same side. Then switch to exhale.

Switch to Exhale. Inhale same side.

Switch to Exhale. Inhale same side.

Switch to Exhale. Inhale same side.

Traditionally, the exhale is longer than the inhale. You could try counting to four as you inhale, another count to hold the air, then eight counts as you exhale. Don't get caught up in the count-

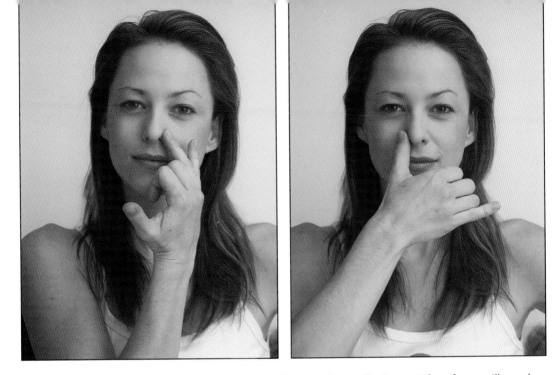

ing though; just go for an easy, long exhale and let the rhythm find you. (After if you still need to count sheep, go right ahead!)

Try this for a few minutes. You might even close the eyes to draw your attention totally inward.

By concentrating so thoroughly on your breath, you'll notice that the mind can't help but slow down. Watching your rhythmic breath becomes as soothing as watching the waves in the ocean. There's no room for distracting thoughts.

Once you feel evened out and calm, gently move your hand away. Sample a few full breaths, letting yourself savor the balanced feeling that alternate nostril breathing creates.

Benefits:

This breath is deeply calming because it balances the hemispheres of the brain. Breathing in this way allows you to "even out" your thoughts to find a steady balance within.

Final Twist

As the torso twists sideways,
The body releases and lengthens,
Softening the Spirit toward sleep.

Lying down, bend your knees, letting your feet come to the mattress.

Swivel your hips a bit over to the left, letting your right bottom cheek stay on the ground, as your left one lifts up a bit.

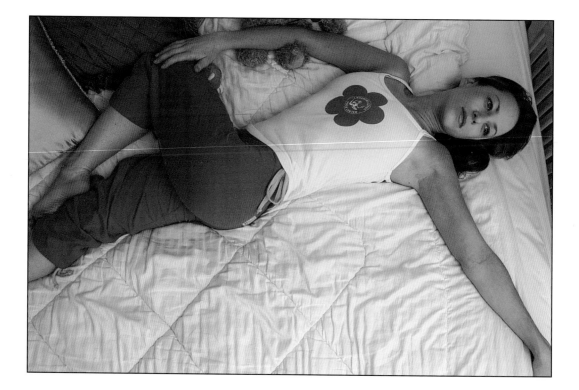

Keeping the hips where they are, draw your left knee towards your chest, and let your leg go long and straight against the mattress.

Gently take the lightly bent left leg over to the right side of the body, letting your right hand come to the top of the thigh. The weight of the hand can gently drift the leg further towards the mattress.

It's more important, however, to keep both shoulders releasing on the mattress. Let the left shoulder open softly on the mattress so that the open palm can reach away. Gently let your head turn towards the open palm, keeping your neck released in the shape.

Keep the shape gentle and relaxed, lingering for a good handful of breaths, perhaps even a minute or more. Let each breath open you more and more.

When you're ready, inhale and come back to neutral.

Then reverse everything for the other side, keeping that same, easy relaxed feeling in the shape.

Benefit:

This sweet twist allows you to let go very deeply, moving you closer and closer to sleep with every breath in it.

Rock-a-bye Roll

Knees snuggled into the chest
Instills the cozy feelings of bedtime
Through the entire psyche.

A repeat of the morning roll.

Draw your knees into your chest, hugging them gently. Find the variation that works for you—either knees together or apart.

If it feels nice to lift the head up into the shape, go ahead—just make sure you don't strain the neck.

Part of the fun of rolling yourself into this compressed ball is that when you release, everything just lets go completely. Any remaining tension in the body knows it's time to take off, as you prepare yourself to drift sweetly off for the night.

Benefits:

Lower back releases as hips loosen. Feelings of ease result.

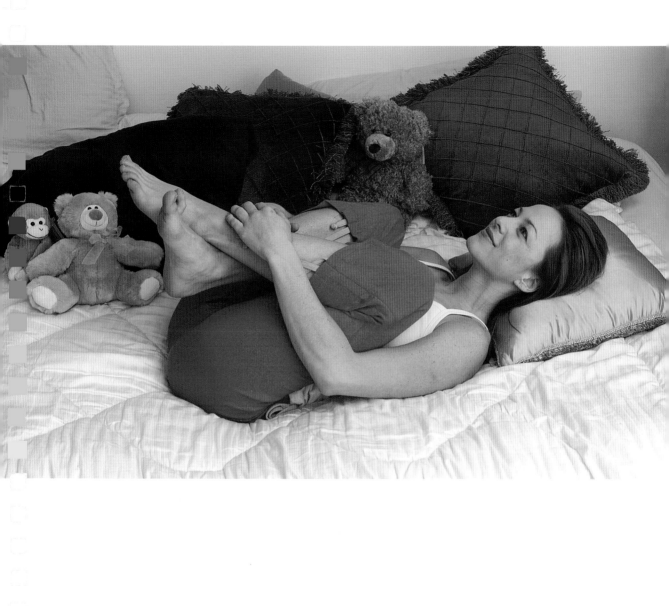

Chill Out Meditation

Chill out completely so
The relaxed mind
Can drift off to dreamland…

You might try this meditation seated or lying down. As always, choose the most comfortable position for you.

Sometimes lying down can be tricky because you might get so relaxed you fall asleep—not that that's a bad thing at bedtime, though! You might even make the intention that you'll use the meditation to relax and then easily drift with a truly carefree mind.

I've found that the key to chilling out is staying present. Too often we're focused on the past or the future. The best way to get centered in the present is to focus on your breath.

Allow your attention to shift to your breathing, watching the inhale and the exhale. Develop an almost X-ray vision to see inside yourself. Once you're feeling connected inside, you can notice how effortlessly your thoughts settle and slow down.

The breath is your most powerful tool in yoga because it not only tells you what your mental state is—rushed and anxious or calm and centered—but also because by changing your breath, you can truly change your state of mind. Even the act of simply observing your breath begins to shape it, calming you and centering your energy.

At the end of your day, it's time to let everything go. Feel gratitude for the blessings in your life but release all the tensions, uncertainties, and things you can't control. Again, the key to this is staying focused in the present moment, precisely where you are right now, living beautifully breath to breath.

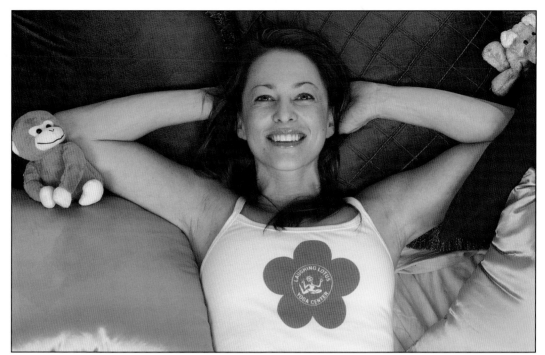

I'm not talking about denial or running away from your problems. Instead, I'm suggesting an open acceptance of where you are. In the morning you have the day in front or you to take charge of things that are within your control, but right now all that's required is that you allow yourself the invaluable gift of sleep.

Beyond working with the breath, how can you learn to let go?

There's no easy answer. Like many things in life, simply being willing to try is the first and biggest step.

The second step might be choosing to focus on something positive—whether it's your breath or your blessings. Otherwise your mind will skip all over the place, lingering on any anxieties even if those can't be improved in the present moment.

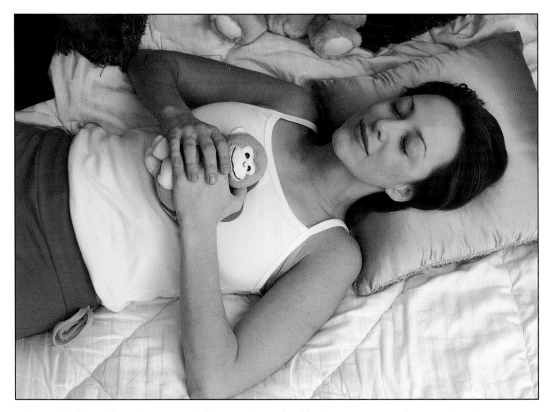

The third step is to keep practicing yoga's path of letting go, accepting, and staying present through poses, breath-work, and meditations. A daily dose of *Yoga in Bed* is certainly a great beginning. Let it become your foundation towards building greater peace of mind. Even on those days when you must leap right out of bed and into the jungle of your life, try to make time for a few moments of meditation and breathing.

I'm not saying it's easy. In fact, as you chill out from your day, even when you practice, you'll probably find that the mind does often get restless. Some meditation experts have compared the mind to a puppy that requires constant, gentle training in order for it to sit still. But ultimately, with practice, like that sweet puppy, it'll get easier and easier to have the mind simply stay put when you want it to. It'll become your faithful friend and not a source of constant distraction.

So right now, as you chill out, be easy on yourself whenever a worry or a concern pops up. Don't let it trouble you. Simply notice whatever's occurring on your mental radar. Without paying too much attention to it, let it drift away with the current of your thoughts.

Indeed, most of our problems are not in the present; they're things we're brooding about that have already happened or imagined things we're stressing over before they even occur. Staying truly present, we find there are far fewer problems, and even those are usually more manageable than we might think. (Some things even work themselves out all by themselves!)

Try to stay steady with your Chill Out Meditation, despite the ever-changing shape of your thoughts. Always your mind will drag you into the past or the future, but bring things back to the present. Just breath.

Rest as long as you like in this Chill Out meditation, either floating directly off to sleep or completing it anyway you like.

Before drifting off, don't forget to congratulate yourself on a successful yoga practice, one that every day makes you freer in your body, more centered in your thoughts, and closer to your heart.

Benefits:

The peace of mind that a Chill Out Meditation brings helps the body as well as the mind. Countless studies demonstrate that calming one's nervous system through steady breathing and centering one's thoughts brings good health and increases personal happiness dramatically.

OM!

Yoga While Asleep

In the Tibetan practice, there is actually a yoga that concentrates on dreams and sleep. It's full of fascinating practices and rituals to allow an individual to become spiritually awakened through dreaming lucidly.

Lucid dreaming has met with increasing interest in the West. Scientists are studying its effects. Beyond this, for centuries people have been studying and working with their dreams as keys to all sorts of insights. Great scientists have sworn that their greatest discoveries appeared through dreams. Many people report uncanny prophetic dreams involving verifiable premonitions. And who hasn't had a dream that had some meaningful effect on his or her life?

You might try recording your dreams and sharing them with a friend. There are many great books on lucid dreaming, so you might try the "Matrix-y" experience of trying to awaken within a dream. It's a fascinating practice and if the Tibetan yogis are right, might just bring you a giant step towards awakening into your spiritual destiny. Sweet dreams indeed!

Make Your Sleep Space Special

It's important to love where you sleep. Try to make your bedroom a place that relaxes and calms you simply by being present in it. When decorating, stay within your budget, but make sure everything suits you and your taste.

First, since you have to have sheets, blankets, and pillows no matter what, try to find ones that please you aesthetically. Put a little thought into the colors, textures, and lighting choices you're making in the space. Even changing a lampshade, or adding a splash of color with throw pillows, can make a huge difference. There are many sources for "cheap decorating tips" that demonstrate that a small can of paint or the right framed poster can transform the feeling of any space.

It's important that the bedroom be conducive to sleep. The right mattress is key, but so is regulating the environment to what feels best for you. An absence of light and loud noises is essential, especially if you live in a bright, noisy city. Find the right window treatments to block out distractions, or try ear plugs or even a soothing white-noise machine.

Climate control counts, too. An appropriate temperature should be maintained so that your body isn't either struggling to stay warm or sweating. Humidifiers or air filters might be necessary as well.

Set the Mood

After you evaluate the comfort level of your bedroom, continue being generous with yourself. Make it a place you love. A great way to do this is to surround yourself with things that please you, whether that's candles or flowers or a picture of your favorite hockey team, or a corny vacation souvenir. If your choices evoke the feelings you want to create around falling asleep easily—calm, centered, happy associations—you're one big step closer to Dreamland.

Keep Your Sleep Space Sacred

You can help make smooth transitions to "sleep mode," by remembering to keep your bedroom as a sacred space, reserved only for sleep (and sex and yoga). This way, you're much more likely to swing into the right mindset when you want. By limiting the uses of your bed, you subconsciously help yourself drift off more easily.

If you can't keep some of your work-life out of the bedroom (perhaps, you are a freelancer living in a studio apartment), try to keep the work itself out of bed. Don't make business calls lying down or read annual reports right before sleeping. If keeping your work and your bed separate is not possible—I have a writer friend who can only work if she brings her laptop into bed and reclines under the covers!—at the end of the day, remove everything and clear the space.

In the same way on a restless night, it's also a good idea not to linger in bed getting more and more frustrated. If you haven't fallen asleep in fifteen or twenty minutes, researchers recommend getting up and doing something else that's soothing, rather than tossing and turning. Occupy your mind with something else other than your inability to doze off, and return to your bed only when you feel tired again.

Evaluate your own bedroom behavior thoroughly to make sure you're creating and preserving your own personal sleep sanctuary.

Make Good Sleep a Priority

Another key element of many rituals is timing. First, give yourself "permission" to go to bed. I know that might sound a little silly, but so often we feel responsible for so many things, that we don't allow ourselves something we truly need, like sleep. There's always another important thing that has to get done and we feel bad or lazy if we're not accomplishing it.

Surveys show that most people will cheat their sleep time in order to get work done without too much thought, and yet study after study demonstrates that a sleepy employee is just not as productive as a well-rested one. So if you're constantly not getting enough sleep because you "don't have time" to sleep, you might want to rethink how you've organized your priorities. Treat yourself to the rest you need!

Standardize Your Bedtime

It's good to have a set time for falling asleep. You don't necessarily need to have as rigid a bedtime (or a curfew) as when you were a kid, but you might want to have a relatively narrow window of when you hit the hay. The more you can standardize when you go to bed, the more easily your body clock can keep to the schedule that works best for you.

In the same way, it's not a great idea to wildly vary your weekend and work week sleep schedules. Your body doesn't know it's Saturday night and time to stay up until 4 AM, but that Sunday night requires you fast asleep by 11 PM so you can beat the morning commute. Of course those special occasions will arise that steal away your sleep time—and who doesn't want to share a spontaneous fun night out with friends on the dance floor—but in general, crazy weekend schedules make your week nights much more difficult to manage.

Opt for Healthy Lifestyle Choices

Many broader lifestyle choices help with successful sleeping.

Exercise is a terrific way to help yourself have sweet, steady dreams. Aside from all the other numerous benefits of working out, studies show that exercising regularly helps tremendously with a good night of sleep. By exercising sensibly, your general health will improve of course, thus helping to avoid many issues associated with troubled sleep.

But again, don't exercise too close to bedtime.

Stimulants like caffeine obviously challenge the relaxation process. Cutting down on coffee or caffeine-filled soda—certainly those consumed in the hours before bedtime—might significantly improve your ability to get to sleep.

Realize, too, that alcohol is *not* helpful as a sleep aide. Although it might make you feel slightly more relaxed, even sometimes a little drowsy, alcohol significantly decreases the quality of your sleep. It's wise to limit alcohol intake right before bed, so that your sleep time doesn't becoming about "sleeping it off."

In addition, over-consumption of food can also impede sleep. While a soothing light bedtime snack might be OK, a big meal before bed probably isn't the best idea. It's not fun to tuck yourself in feeling bloated and heavy.

Finally, when it comes to sleep wisdom, smoking is another big "no no." Studies show that smokers not only take longer to fall asleep, but also wake up more often during the night. Beyond that, it doesn't facilitate yoga, given all the emphasis on breathing in yoga.

Getting Good in Bed

In summary, so many of the things we equate with healthy living—such as exercising regularly and having a routine, while avoiding smoking or excessive drinking—are also the things that contribute to the quality of our sleep. Study after study shows that these healthy habits reflect good sleep, and vice versa: good sleep yields a healthier you.

So if you're having trouble sleeping, look to these areas in your life, seeing if you can fine-tune them and create a more pleasant nightly visit to dreamland.

Overcoming Insomnia and Other Sleep Disorders_____

Over 40 million Americans suffer from sleep disorders, affecting a higher percentage of women. In fact 53 percent of women aged 30–60 experience difficulty sleeping often or always. Yet strangely, only 41 percent of women think they have insomnia in the past year, meaning that a sound night's sleep is no longer expected.

Many factors can affect one's sleep, including depression, stress, anxiety, pain, and general health concerns. So if you're experiencing any problems associated with getting regular, healthy sleep, it's important to consult your physician.

You might also explore information available from these sources:

National Sleep Foundation
1552 K Street, N.W., Suite 500
Washington, DC 20005
202•347•3471
www.sleepfoundation.org

National Center on Sleep Disorder Research
P.O. Box 30105
Bethesda, MD 20824
301•435•0199
www.nhlbi.nih.gov/about/ncsdr